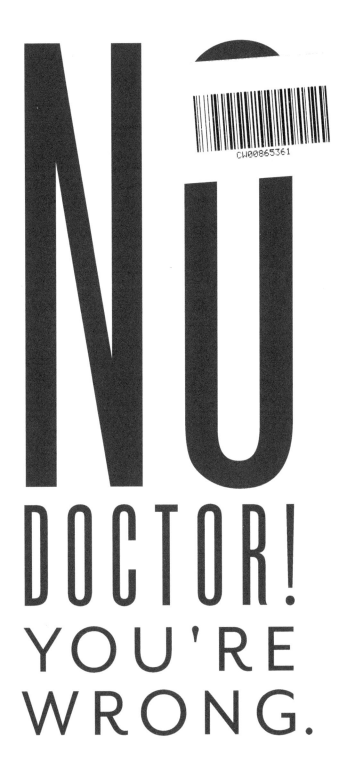

CW00865361

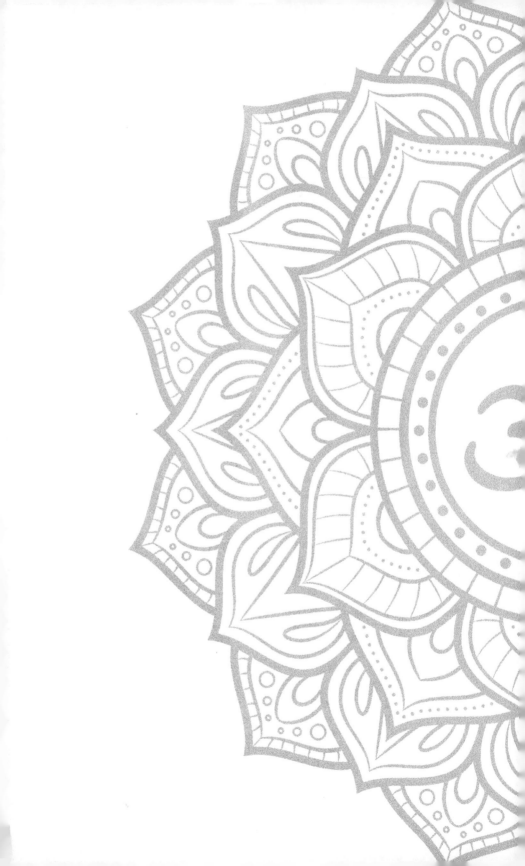

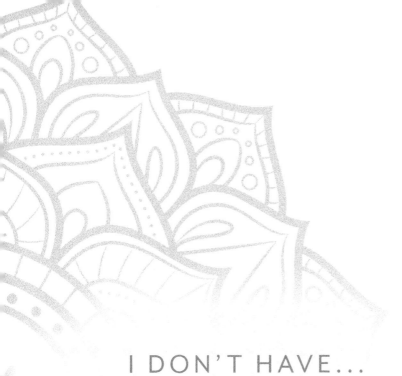

I DON'T HAVE…

How My Husband Saved My Life When I Was
Misdiagnosed Over and Over and Over…..

SHERRI ANTOINETTE

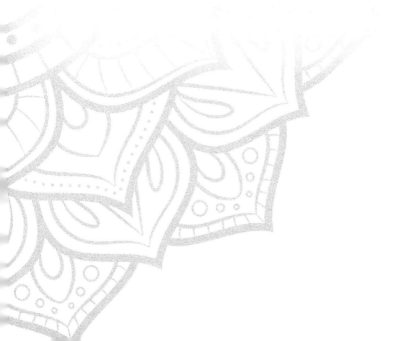

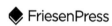

Suite 300 - 990 Fort St
Victoria, BC, V8V 3K2
Canada

www.friesenpress.com

ISBN
978-1-5255-6433-8 (Hardcover)
978-1-5255-6434-5 (Paperback)
978-1-5255-6435-2 (eBook)

1. BIOGRAPHY & AUTOBIOGRAPHY, MEDICAL

Distributed to the trade by The Ingram Book Company

A physical,
emotional,
and spiritual journey
from dis-ease to healing

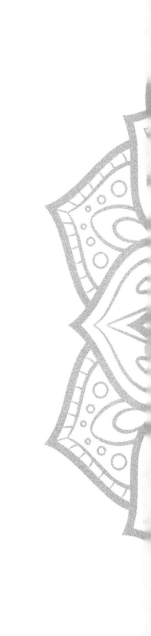

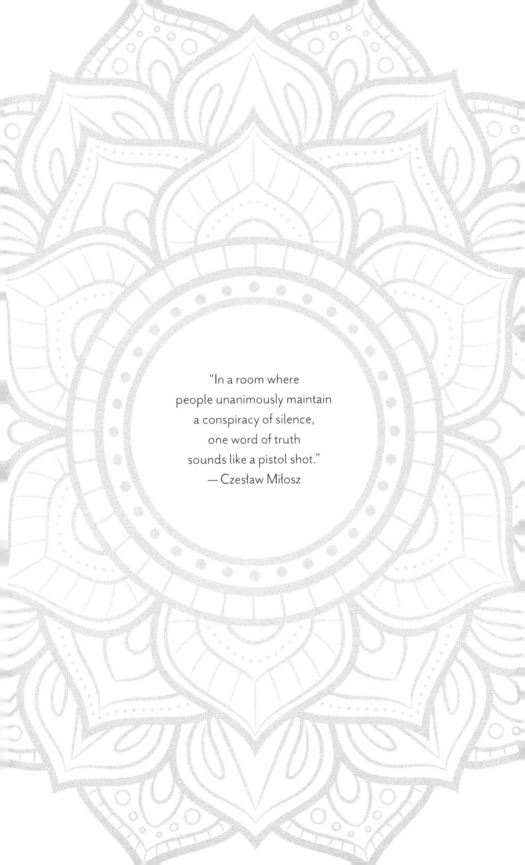

"In a room where
people unanimously maintain
a conspiracy of silence,
one word of truth
sounds like a pistol shot."
— Czesław Miłosz

DEDICATION

I dedicate this book to William, the love of my life! If not for your perseverance, love, and commitment, I would probably not be here, or I would be unable to use my fingers to type or my brain to organize the words in this book. You gave me the strength and courage not only to survive the dis-ease that ravaged my body but to rise above it and share my experiences. I will be forever grateful for your abiding belief that the medical doctors' diagnoses were wrong, and that "if it is the last thing you ever do," you "would find what my issue was and fix it." Your love has saved me more times than you would ever know. Thank you for being on this journey with me, through the tears, the doubt, the heartache, and the pain. Thank you for supporting me in the writing of this book without knowing the title or reading even one word of it!

I searched my heart for words to express all you have been to me, but nothing I came up with seemed to be enough. As I thought about what I wanted to say, this song by Celine Dion popped into my head, and to you, William, the love of my life, I say:

> For all those times you stood by me
> For all the truth that you made me see
> For all the joy you brought to my life
> For all the wrong that you made right
> For every dream you made come true
> For all the love I found in you
> I'll be forever thankful, baby
> You're the one who held me up
> Never let me fall
> You're the one who saw me through, through it all

You gave me wings; you made me fly
You touched my hand; I could touch the sky
I lost my faith; you gave it back to me
You said no star was out of reach
You stood by me, and I stood tall
I had your love; I had it all
I'm grateful for each day you gave me
Maybe I don't know that much
But I know this much is true
I am blessed because I am loved by you

You were always there for me
The tender wind that carried me
A light in the dark, shining your love into my life
You've been my inspiration
Through the lies, you were the truth
My world is a better place because of you

You were my strength when I was weak
You were my voice when I couldn't speak
You were my eyes when I couldn't see
You saw the best there was in me
Lifted me up, when I couldn't reach
You gave me faith, 'cause you believed
I'm everything I am
BECAUSE YOU LOVE ME!

I love you to the moon and back, infinity and beyond.
Forever and ever, amen!

I also dedicate this book to my mother, the first love of my life! You planted the seed of hope in me, despite your hopelessness, and you made me believe that I am worthy of love and respect. Thank you for protecting me, and thank you for teaching me about courage by the things you did and, sometimes, more importantly, didn't do. If you asked me to, I would do it all over again because I love you unconditionally! I dedicate this poem I used to write in your homemade Mother's Day card when I was a child, to you. I think of you every single day, and I am at peace knowing you've found your peace and happiness. You are only a thought away because you live in my heart, and our love transcends all physical boundaries. I love you, Mom!

M… is for the million things you gave me
O… means only that you're growing old
T… is for the tears you shed to save me
H… is for your heart of purest gold
E… is for your eyes with loves' light shining
R… means right and right you'll always be

Put them all together they spell MOTHER,
A word that means the world to me!

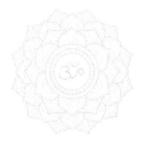

TABLE OF CONTENTS

INTRODUCTION

T hank you for taking the time to read this book. It is with great appreciation and gratitude that I offer my humble opinions, which I base on personal experiences. I developed some kind of physical ailment that stopped my life dead in its tracks, and when I sought help from the medical community, they didn't believe I was unwell or diagnosed me with diseases I knew were wrong. My journey to getting to a diagnosis is one I never thought I would be on because I just wanted someone to tell me what was physically wrong with me so I could fix it.

My reason for sharing my story is that, all through the pain and misdiagnoses, I kept thinking to myself, *there is no way I am the only one in the world with this problem.* I hope that, if I am not, people who develop physical symptoms like I had will have doctors who listen to them and find their issues, hopefully preventing months or years of pain and suffering. For those of you who are getting diagnoses that do not resonate with you, I hope you continue to push to find out what is truly wrong. Don't accept a diagnosis that will ultimately lead to suffering and a 'premature' end.

I've shared some deeply personal stories, memories I tried to suppress for over forty years. As I lived through my ordeal and learned what I did, I realized there were many facets to my condition that needed to be understood and resolved. I believe with all my heart that dis-ease in the body has an emotional component way before it manifests itself physically. I use this word dis-ease, not in the conventional meaning of a disease, but to mean my body is not at ease. I want to shine a light on the possibility that, when a disease finally does manifest in the body, we view it from a physical, emotional, *and* spiritual perspective, and not deal only with the physicality of it.

I share my story to give **hope** to anyone who is experiencing a physical ailment and has been misdiagnosed or told nothing is wrong. I hope I can provoke thought about the effects of a prolonged, unhealthy emotional state on the body and the potential for a physical disease to manifest. This hope can also relate to those who are dealing with emotional trauma, as I offer a spiritual perspective of looking at life experiences. These are just my perspectives, garnered from my experiences, and are what got me through the toughest times and thoughts. I believe that, if I didn't have the perspectives I did, it would have surely ended in disaster.

I wish you well if you are on a journey from dis-ease to healing. Never give up hope, and you, too, will find the answers!

DIS-EASE

am lying on the examination table in the Nuclear Medicine Department of the local hospital. After I changed into the gown the nurse gave me, I did as she asked and awaited her return. It is a few months before my fiftieth birthday, and I am about to have a bone scan. The machine above me looks larger than life and a bit menacing, and even though I know it's a helpful tool, it still scares me. It stands over and around me and looks like it will engulf my very soul. Maybe it's not the machine at all; perhaps it's just what it could find that's scary—the potential culprit: cancer.

I fight the thought, *What if?* The room is cold, and I struggle to stop shaking. The trembling is partly because of fear; this thing could find that I have a disease in my body that could change the course of my life. Intuitively, I feel I don't have cancer, but what if? What if I'm in denial? I shake my head as if to get rid of the thoughts and assure myself they are premature and unnecessary and are causing anxiety—I have to calm down.

The nurse comes and has a lovely bedside manner, which puts me at ease. I am glad because anyone staring up at this almost threatening-looking machine is here for a potentially horrible reason. She explains that she will take images of different parts of my body, and she will instruct me on what to do each time. She talks me through the process and does several scans, and it takes approximately twenty minutes.

I got dressed and left the room and headed out to my waiting husband, William. I've been in this hospital before, and this was not my first test.

By that time, I'd had blood tests and CT scans of my chest, abdomen, and pelvis. A question kept circulating in my head: *How did I end up here?*

I've had symptoms for thirteen months, and gotten diagnoses I believed were incorrect but cancer? In April of 2017, I noticed my fingers on both hands were warm and tingling. I was a bit concerned, since both my parents had diabetes and passed from complications from the disease, my mother only three weeks earlier.

I had seen my family doctor a couple of weeks before, for my regular annual visit, and had said, "See you next year," which was our running joke when we saw each other once a year. I was a bit concerned about this tingling and thought I had to check it out because of my family history with diabetes. Even though my mother had diabetes, she'd never had this particular symptom, but I was still concerned.

I didn't necessarily believe I was doomed to have diabetes, just because both my parents did because I had lived a different life. I was a borderline vegetarian, exercised five days a week, didn't drink alcohol or smoke, and had been on a spiritual journey over the last few years, practicing mindfulness and meditation.

Not long after the tingling in my hands started, I developed pain in my left side and decided it was time to go back to the doctor, as there was no relief.

When he saw me, he said, "What are you doing here? I saw you a few weeks ago."

After laughing about him not saying, long time no see and me responding with don't take it personally, that's a good thing, I described the pain to him as a stitch. It was neither sharp nor dull but somewhere in the middle—a constant sensation that felt like I had run too far too fast, and got an awful stitch. I explained that it wouldn't budge no matter how I stretched or moved.

I also mentioned the tingling fingers and expressed my concern about diabetes. My doctor examined my stomach area, feeling for whatever doctors feel for, and he ordered blood work, a pelvic ultrasound, and a colonoscopy, as he suspected diverticulitis. He was sure there was nothing to worry about and said that, if it were diverticulitis, I would have a round of antibiotics and be fine.

His assistant Christy was very efficient and got me a colonoscopy appointment in a relatively short time. I was nervous at this appointment and the process since I'd never had the procedure. I remembered my doctor saying there was nothing to be nervous about, as drinking the solution to clean out the intestines probably was worse than the procedure itself.

I breathed a sigh of relief when all the tests came back negative. I was not diabetic or even prediabetic, as my sugar levels were perfect. I didn't have diverticulitis, and my pelvic ultrasound was negative for any issues. The stitch, by this time, seemed to be intensifying, and over-the-counter (OTC) pain meds were of no help.

One night, as I relaxed in bed, just before dozing off, I noticed my heart rate was very deep and loud—so loud that I could hear and feel it pounding in my ears as well as in my jaw. I thought it was strange since one is not supposed to hear their heart beating, especially when relaxed in bed. I tried to ignore it, but it was difficult since it seemed to rock me. It felt as if my heart was also in my stomach of all places, and I figured I was getting anxious about my symptoms and just needed to not think about them and go to sleep.

My stitch got worse, and my alarm bells were going off because the pain was not only on my left but had now spread to my right side, and it felt like something was squeezing my stomach. The sensation reminded me of when I got my blood pressure taken, that squeezing sensation that almost feels like pain, but the doctor stops just short of causing pain and releases the air, so there is relief.

I went back to my family doctor, this time, to let him know about the pounding heart. I also told him I had developed very itchy legs, which seemed to get itchier when I scratched. He pulled one side of his trousers up to his knee and scratched his legs to show me his dry skin, and I did the same, only my scratches did not leave white marks like his did. I told him of the pounding heart and how it was uncomfortable and affected my ability to fall asleep. I mentioned that I was probably premenopausal because I was nearing my forty-ninth birthday.

He said that my blood vessels were clogged, and this caused the pounding sensation and explained that even though it might feel as though it was harder for my heart to pump blood, it wasn't working harder than normal. His explanation made no sense to me, and he didn't order any tests to confirm that my arteries were clogged. I understood that it was just something I had to endure, even though it affected my ability to fall asleep.

As for my stitch, he diagnosed me with Irritable Bowel Syndrome (IBS), since none of the testing I had done up to that point showed any cause for concern. This diagnosis did not resonate with me since I had no ongoing digestive issues. I discovered on my own that being on the pill may have resulted in a magnesium deficiency, and after taking calcium/magnesium supplements, I was okay. Before finding the potential link between magnesium deficiency and constipation, I mentioned to my family doctor that my diet couldn't be responsible for my condition. I knew it wasn't because I made sure to eat high-fiber foods such as bran flakes, prunes, salads, whole grains, and so on, which didn't help at all. To alleviate my constipation, he prescribed some thick orange liquid, which didn't work. About my premenopausal suspicions, he didn't agree and said I should stay on the pill.

I expressed my concern about having been on a synthetic hormone for over twenty-eight years, and he told me his "sister is still on it, and she's sixty-five." A bit thrown by this tidbit, which had no relevance to me, I wasn't going to argue the potential risks of staying on this medication, as I had already decided to stop taking it. It was not something I wanted to use, but he had prescribed it in my early twenties as a way to deal with terrible menstrual issues and horrible acne.

I also wanted to know if my body had begun this inevitable life change, as there had been signs for about two years, although I didn't realize it at the time. I'd had night sweats for two years prior, but being on the pill ensured that I had a period at the end of every twenty-eight-day cycle. When I had the night sweats, I blamed my poor William, because he always felt like a furnace and I thought sleeping next to him was causing me to sweat during the night.

I left my doctor's office for the second time, none the wiser about what was happening to my body, but I knew in my gut (no pun intended) that I did not have IBS. I researched it, and I didn't have the same symptoms.

There was no ongoing constipation, diarrhea, nausea, or any other related symptom, just the stitch, and nothing I ate aggravated the pain. William and I often joke that I am the one with guts of steel.

A month later, with no relief in sight, I went to the doctor who was looking after my family doctor's patients while he was on vacation. I hoped that maybe this doctor would look at my symptoms with fresh eyes, and we would finally figure it out. If I had known what the outcome was going to be, I would've just stayed home and nursed my pain. The doctor showed me the results of all my previous tests on his computer and said I had a functional disease. I asked what this was, and I don't remember what he said because I was more focused on his tone than on the substance of what was said.

He said that all the results of my blood work, ultrasound, and colonoscopy were fine, and there was nothing wrong with me. I made a joke, partly to get a reaction from him and to confirm in my mind what I thought he was thinking and trying to convey to me. I said, "It seems like I need to see a psychologist."

He didn't respond, but it was more what he didn't say than what he did. He looked at me with a sort of facial expression that said, you said it, I didn't. As much as I don't read minds, I could feel this doctor's attitude toward me, which conveyed that there was nothing wrong with me, so why was I in his office?

When I got home, I googled functional disease. The first hit from Wikipedia states that a functional disease is a medical condition that impairs the normal functioning of bodily processes that remains largely undetected under examination, dissection, or even under a microscope. At the exterior, there is no appearance of abnormality.[1] If this didn't confuse me even more, I didn't know what would have.

Where do I go with a diagnosis like this, and what do I take for the pain? These three doctor visits sent me on a trajectory filled with excruciating pain and many failed attempts to deal with it, including emergency room visits and multiple wrong diagnoses that made me question my mental health. These misdiagnoses led me down a path of suicidal thoughts, spiritual exploration, and doubting my faith in something bigger than myself because the pain was so unbearable. It taught me the power of my mind and spirit when I was able to control the negative thoughts I had when the pain was so bad that all I wanted was to die.

It was an experience that taught me how to deal with the loss of my independence, as I was unable to take care of myself. It showed me what love is when my partner and love of my life never gave up on me, even when I gave up on myself. It taught me about a type of love I did not know existed or was possible because it was not something I had seen in relationships as I was growing up.

THE SEARCH CONTINUES...

realized I was not going to get any answers from the conventional medical doctors I had seen up to that point, and thought I would try another route. Seeking the help of a naturopath seemed like my only recourse because no matter which medical doctor I went to, based on seemingly random symptoms at this point—my stitch, tingling fingers, itchy legs, and pounding heart—they could not or would not help me. Who knows what other diagnoses were around the corner?

I figured maybe a fresh pair of eyes, not trained in the conventional way, would be able to see something that others had missed. I had turned forty-nine by this point, yet I never felt like I was forty-nine. I had always looked younger than my age, and most of the time, I felt it too. I was still able to do between three and three and a half miles on my treadmill five times a week, and I was in a healthy relationship with someone who treated me with love and respect. We ate healthy, enjoying a fast-food treat from time to time. I was meditating, and my life was relatively stress-free, from my perspective. All I had were these symptoms, which I didn't know what to do with, especially with no guidance from either of the two doctors I had seen.

Desperation is something that makes any logically thinking person make choices they would probably not normally make. I was no exception, and I followed the advice of Dr. Candy, the naturopath. She told me I needed to do a bio-cellular cleanse, and the desperation made me not ask questions but blindly purchase five different naturopathic medications, hoping this would get rid of my pain.

Dr. Candy said that my body was toxic, and I needed to do a cleanse to rid my body of these toxins. I couldn't understand how toxins could result in such a specific kind of constant pain. I explained all my test results to her at the initial consultation, which cost $240 an hour.

She recommended that I keep a food journal for two weeks, but, at the end of the time, she really couldn't tell me to do anything differently, as it seemed to her I ate healthily. After about six weeks of this bio-cellular cleanse and a couple more visits at $170 an hour, nothing changed. I kept the IBS diagnosis at the back of my mind, and William suggested that I get off gluten to see if this made a difference. I tried a gluten-free diet for over a month, but the pain continued to get worse.

Auricular medicine was Dr. Candy's specialty, and because I believe there are all kinds of healing modalities that work for a variety of issues, I was open to trying anything. But, when she said I needed a different round of the bio-cellular meds after the first gave no relief, that's where I had to draw the line since I had an intuitive feeling that this was not the path for me.

She suggested I do an allergy test to see if there were any foods I was allergic to, but this seemed unnecessary since my food journal showed no red flags. I did a food allergy test on my own, and the results showed that I was allergic to apples and hare. I laughed because I never had any sort of reaction on the rare occasion I had an apple. The last time I ate hare (actually, it was rabbit) was in 1990 when a friend at university made it, and I'd had no adverse reaction to it then.

Dr. Candy didn't do any other testing, except to use a machine to test the energy of the supplements I had been taking for years, which were a multi-vitamin, vitamin D, calcium and magnesium, and fish-oil supplements. The idea that I had so much toxicity in my body that required more cleansing made me a bit doubtful of the treatment.

She suggested I use an antihistamine for the crazy itchiness I had on my stomach, which I believe was a premenopausal symptom, and it helped, but I still had itchy legs. I tried to alleviate the itching on my legs by changing laundry detergents, and I also stopped using dryer sheets. I started using a showerhead filter and changed my body lotions. Nothing seemed to quell the never-ending itch on my legs. I abandoned this attempt to go natural, as I wondered how many more of these cleanses I had to do to be toxin-free.

Nothing I ate seemed to irritate my digestive system or impact the pain. By this time, however, it seemed like the pain got worse when I did any twisting, bending, or any general movement of my torso. I was still able to walk on the treadmill, but it dwindled to twenty minutes.

By October, the stitch like pain had gotten so much worse, and it started to affect the way I moved my body. Washing my hair became a basic hygiene task fraught with anxiety because when I raised my arms to wash my hair, the stitch in my sides felt like it was tightening up so much it brought tears to my eyes.

It was not only raising my arms that made the stitch get progressively worse but any movement at all. It didn't matter what I did, bending over, reaching for something; anything that entailed movement of my torso felt like a blood pressure cuff was squeezing around my waist. The pain now felt like a gas pain had married the worse cramp I ever had and was now in the solar plexus region of my stomach, and I decided to seek the help of medical doctors again.

I visited my local emergency room on a cool October morning because the pain felt different, and it scared me. I didn't know what was happening to my body, and I was afraid that something would erupt inside me. I thought by the time this happened, and doctors figured out what was wrong, it would be too late. It took an hour before I saw a doctor, which I was ecstatic about (since the usual wait times in this ER were over six hours). Little did I know that this was only the beginning of an ordeal that would last much, much longer.

The ER doctor examined my stomach and asked the usual questions regarding bowel movements and diet. I told him that I'd had the best poop that morning and had no constipation or diarrhea. He gave me a cocktail of pills and a blue liquid and said it would help with the pain, and he ordered blood work. He didn't say what he was expecting to find, and I didn't ask, thinking the only blood work I previously had was to check for diabetes, so maybe he was onto something.

Sitting in the waiting room, watching my fellow patients with varying types of pain with different issues, some crying, made me feel even worse. Some of them had been waiting even longer than me by my fourth hour. I observed the doctors' body language and felt anger and compassion for them at the same time. There were mothers with crying babies in the hallway, but the doctors walked by and wouldn't make eye contact with them.

Even though the patients were seen at some point, I still felt angry because I assumed that they felt as ignored as I did. Then a wave of compassion for the medical staff came over me. I reminded myself that they work twelve-hour shifts with sick people who were sometimes abusive, and being in this kind of environment couldn't be easy. Yet I couldn't help but think that it was their choice to be there, so they should be more empathetic.

The reality of the situation was that they were only human, and there was only so much emotion they could share in the stressful environment in which they worked. That was my way of dealing with what seemed like coldness on their part. Even though the wait time seemed unavoidable, a passing glance to say, I see you, and I know you've been waiting a long time, but we can't help it, would've gone a long way.

It took almost four hours to get the results of my blood work and another hour to see the doctor for the results. He finally gave me the news that nothing was wrong. When I asked what he had looked for in the blood test, he said that, sometimes, heart issues mask themselves as digestive problems or stomach pain. He ordered a CT scan, and I never saw him again. I waited another three hours for the CT scan, partly because I had to drink water and wait a while, but mostly it was just the wait time for a scan.

I was shuffled from one examination room to the next, depending on what procedure was needed, and back to the waiting area. I tried to think of being anywhere else but there, as I sat near the nurses' station, people watching, and my heart just went out to my fellow patients, who by my standards were worse off than I was (or so I convinced myself). The crying babies were the worst to observe, as they seemed so helpless, and I didn't mind if they were attended to before I was. I hadn't eaten since breakfast, and I was famished but couldn't leave the area for fear the results would come back, and I would lose my chance to speak to a doctor.

I saw the relative of a lady who was in a wheelchair and wailing about her pain, starting to get aggressive. He was angry because it seemed no one cared about helping his partner, who was obviously in dire discomfort. The staff reaction to his behavior was to warn him about his language, and when he wouldn't back down, they just ignored him. I thought to myself that getting mad wouldn't help the situation, and as much as I felt like shouting too, I realized it was better to deal with the frustration silently.

I asked if I could go home and have someone contact me regarding my test results, and the nurse said I had to wait to see a doctor. By this time, I was so frustrated and hungry that I couldn't help myself and felt the tears rolling down my face. I was not really in any more pain than when I'd come in, around eleven that morning, but by 10:00 p.m., it had taken its toll.

Being shuffled from one examination room to the next, lugging around my stuff, and trying to ignore the hunger in my belly caught up to me, and the frustration got to a boiling point.

Two ER doctors I saw milling about, finally came with the results of my CT scan and gave me the good news. There was no blockage they could see, and everything looked fine. They diagnosed me with IBS and recommended I go on the FODMAP diet. I was too tired and hungry to ask what this was, and since Google had become my best friend over the last few months, I just thanked them. It was now after midnight, and I just wanted to get out of the hospital.

As I started to get dressed, I couldn't find my pants! In moving around from room to room, they seemed to have disappeared. I'm sure it was not as warm out as it had been when I first came in that morning, but I had to leave the hospital in the gown I was wearing. As I maneuvered my way through the maze of hospital hallways toward the exit, all I could think about was somebody accosting me, thinking I was a runaway patient or to say I couldn't leave with their property. No one did, and I made a mad dash for the car. I was lucky the weather was not that cold for October because my car was parked halfway across the parking lot.

As I was driving home, I started laughing as I asked myself, *Who loses their pants in a hospital?* I was trying to find some humor or something to make me feel better about the last thirteen hours in the ER, which had yielded nothing. It didn't last very long, and I had to fight back the tears because I couldn't see when the oncoming vehicles' lights shone in my eyes.

I was back at square one, no closer to an explanation about what was happening to me than I had been thirteen hours ago. I still didn't believe I had IBS because I did not show the kind of symptoms associated with the disease.

The more you try not to think about something, the more you think about it. If I said, don't think of a purple elephant, that's the thought that would come to mind. That was my experience with this awful pain. As hard as I tried to ignore it, there it was with every movement, day in and day out, and by the end of November, it was starting to take a toll on me mentally.

I kept trying different kinds of OTC topical and oral pain medications, with no ease, and there was nothing I could do about the pounding heartbeat. We usually go away over the Christmas holidays, so I focused on our impending trip and looked forward to the ten or so days where at least the lovely beaches and warm weather could distract me. As much as I was in pain, I tried to persuade myself that it wasn't getting that much worse and thought that maybe, one day, I would wake up and it would just be gone.

On a Sunday morning in late November, I decided to be lazy and stay in bed since William had a Christmas work event to attend. I felt mentally drained from the pain, and it was my 'down weekend' (the weekend I had my period), so I thought I would just laze around.

Out of nowhere, a headache hit me, the likes of which I had never felt before, and I could swear I heard a loud bang. I thought to myself, *What fresh new hell is this!?*

This pain was different! I had suffered seasonal migraines for a few years, but over the past couple of winters, they seemed to ease a bit. I instantly thought; *This is not a migraine!* I knew a migraine, and this was something far more diabolical. The pain emanated from my jaw and neck area and went up the back of my head and to my forehead. It was so bad that even turning my head made it feel like it would implode. The agonizing pain also radiated from inside both ears, but especially the left one, and across the back of my head. I couldn't even get off the bed to get something for the pain or to get my phone to call William to say that something was wrong. Part of me didn't want to, since I'd been sick since April and didn't want to ruin his time out since he was also going through the experience with me.

I'd never really let on how much pain I was in up until this point because I didn't want to add more stress to the already stressful situation of not knowing what was wrong. I stayed in bed until he got home that evening and found me just where he'd left me hours before. This type of pain was new, and I couldn't understand for the life of me why my body was doing this. It was at this point when I had my first dance with the thought of being dead.

I kept thinking that if I were dead, I wouldn't feel this pain or any other for that matter. I quickly tried to think of something else, but I admit that the relief I thought I would get from being dead was appealing. Trying to stay as still as possible was the only recourse at that moment, knowing I would have to move eventually. I told William, after the fact, that maybe it was a good thing I couldn't get out of bed. If I could've, maybe, just maybe, I would have ended it all because this new hell and the last six months had done me in.

The following Monday, I went to my local dentist, because my jaw had locked up. My teeth clenched together, and I couldn't open my mouth but an inch or so. The pain was excruciating, and all I kept thinking was, *What now?*

I felt like my body, which I had taken such good care of over the years by eating healthy and exercising, was now giving up on me. What a waste of time it all was! I had done everything right, and yet, I had spent six months in pain with an explanation I knew was wrong, and now this!

The dentist examined my teeth and said, "There is nothing wrong with your teeth."

Through my clenched jaw, with my vision blurred from the tears in my eyes, I said, "I know there is nothing wrong with my teeth, but I can't open my mouth." My inside voice almost said *Captain Obvious* out loud.

He couldn't help me and referred me to a specialist who could see me the next day. Through the pain, I'd heard him say something about TMJ (temporomandibular joint) disorder, and I knew I wouldn't last another day waiting to see a specialist. I remembered that I'd often seen a sign, as I drove by a shopping plaza, with those same letters, and I heard a voice say, "Go straight there." I've always had strong intuition, not that I listened to it all the time, but this time I was in so much pain that I didn't ignore it. I walked into Dr. Adam's dental office in tears, barely able to talk, and felt lucky because he would see me without an appointment. I only had to wait for about twenty minutes or so to see the dentist.

As I sat in the waiting room, there was a slideshow running on their TV, and I just happened to look up at the moment the 'symptoms of TMJ' were listed on the screen. One of those was tingling in the fingers. If I could've opened my mouth, my jaw would have dropped in shock because who would think tingling fingers had anything to do with jaw issues. I felt a sense of relief and excitement now, thinking this was probably my issue. The dental assistant did X-rays and specialized scans I'd never had before. Then, a TENS (transcutaneous electrical nerve stimulation) machine was applied to my face, jaw, and neck to 'unlock' my jaw. The pain was unlike anything I'd ever felt, but by the end of the three-hour ordeal, Dr. Adam told me I had TMJ disorder.

He explained that grinding or clenching my teeth during sleep may have caused my condition. As well, I'd had 'extra' teeth (I called them riders) removed when I was a young teen. Dr. Adam said these extractions left an imbalance in the structure of my jaw, which caused it to try to find an optimal position, which it attempted to accomplish by clenching.

He said I had to remove all of my wisdom teeth at some point, but immediately, the bottom two, which had never posed a problem before. Dr. Adam made a temporary device to put between my upper and lower teeth to prevent me from further grinding them and to take the pressure off of the temporomandibular joint. He measured my mouth for an orthotic I would wear for three or four months and have it adjusted once a week. The idea was to very gradually bring the bottom jaw, which had dropped to the right, back into alignment with my upper jaw. It seemed simple enough! A mold was made of my bottom teeth to make the orthotic.

I asked Dr. Adam about the connection between TMJ disorder and tingling fingers because I could not wrap my brain around what one had to do with the other. He explained, via a simple song we learned in primary school, that "The hip bone's connected to the..." well, you get the gist. He said the temporomandibular joint has muscles and nerves connected to it and those connected to muscles and nerves in the neck, which connected to nerves in the arms, which run down to the fingers and can cause tingling. I mentioned the stitch like feeling I'd had since April, and my experience trying to figure out what was causing it. He said that it might all have been related since the human body is so interconnected.

At this point, it seemed like all my problems would soon be over with the orthotic, and all I had to do for all to be well was wear it for three or four months and get it adjusted once a week. Since we had found the culprit responsible for so much pain and discomfort, and it seemed an easy fix, we booked our annual Christmas getaway. I had my wisdom teeth removed in early December, and I had a week to recover. Soon, we would be in sunny Jamaica, looking forward to the New Year with the hope that all the pain I had endured for almost eight months would soon be a horrible and distant memory.

While sitting on the beach, enjoying the pleasant smell of the salty air and listening to the waves crash on the shore, I suddenly felt a strange sensation wash over my skin. I had been taking antibiotics and pain meds after the extractions, and all seemed to be going well. The winds were always pretty intense on this particular beach we were at, which is why we liked being there. It kept us cool and kept the cigarette smoke of our fellow beachgoers moving. The winds picked up a bit, and I found myself hiding under my towel because it felt like the blowing wind and sand were assaulting me. It got to be too much, so we relocated to another beach with a calmer breeze.

Thinking nothing of it, we continued to enjoy our time together in the sun, knowing there were snowstorms back home. Then, my left hand started to hurt as if someone was stabbing it. I thought that maybe it was an arthritic pain, since I'd had a work-related repetitive sprain injury years before, and from time to time, I got pains in my hand. I convinced myself that's what it was and had a somewhat enjoyable vacation, despite the pain. I thought all of this would soon end, so it felt easier to endure.

When we got back from Jamaica, I noticed from my pictures that I seemed to have lost some weight. I was able to maintain a healthy weight of between 135 and 140 pounds for most of my adult life, so I wasn't trying to lose weight. I considered this a good thing because who doesn't want to lose a few pounds? And I must admit, I looked good in my bikini.

At my follow-up appointment at the end of January, Dr. Adam installed the orthotic onto my bottom teeth. It was painful having my mouth open for so long, but William stood by my side through the entire process, holding onto my foot. I kept glancing in his direction, looking for some acknowledgment, and in his eyes, I realized I was not the only one in pain. Sometimes, seeing a loved one in pain is just as hard as experiencing pain first hand. He didn't have to say the words, but I understood from his eyes that, though it wasn't physical, he too was experiencing pain.

I tried my best not to show how uncomfortable this procedure was, and as he held onto my foot, I could *feel* him say, I'm here; you will be okay. I tried to be strong because I knew how much he worried about me, and it was calming to feel his warm hand on my foot, encouraging me to stay focused. Dr. Adam was as gentle as he could be under the circumstances and told me what he would do before he did it, preparing me every step of the way.

He said the nerves and muscles connected to the temporomandibular joint had to be retrained into a new position all over again, but the process had to be subtle and not cause more pain. Getting used to this foreign object in my mouth took some time, as I couldn't eat anything hard or bite anything and pull with my teeth. Food is one of my life's pleasures—not that I ate a whole lot, but I loved food and ate whatever I wanted.

You know how sometimes you get something tiny, like a sesame seed, stuck in your teeth, and it feels like a rock? The way the orthotic felt in my mouth was a hundred times worse! It was so uncomfortable and affected what I ate and how I ate, but there was no other choice. The headaches never went away, even though they subsided from the initial day I went in. With every adjustment of the orthotic, there were accompanying headaches and jaw pain.

I made my weekly visits to Dr. Adam's office to have the orthotic adjusted, and, as the weeks went by, the stitch in my sides got increasingly worse. The headaches didn't ease up altogether, and the pain in my neck and back was worsening. I spent days lying on the couch because I could barely move to do much else. The most I was able to do, maybe every few days, was to make a meal. Household chores like vacuuming were now more difficult because my arms were now affected (especially the left one).

I couldn't understand why things were getting worse when they were supposed to be getting better. I asked Dr. Adam about other cases similar to mine, and he said that usually when someone has this issue, they get relief within forty-eight hours and definitely two weeks after installing the orthotic. It had been almost two and a half months since I'd had mine in at this point, and I had not gotten the intended relief.

Since the original plan was to wear the orthotic for three to four months, we thought it best to try to get to that point and take it from there. I spoke to a different hygienist than the one who usually assisted Dr. Adam on my visits, and asked her about her experience with patients with TMJ disorder. I was looking for some yardstick by which to measure my progress or lack thereof. She told me about a patient who had come to their office in a wheelchair because of it, which I took as a sign that I should give it more time.

Still, I wondered how it is that TMJ disorder could cause someone to end up in a wheelchair. I had a hard time understanding how a dysfunction in a joint in one's jaw could result in something as drastic as being unable to walk. But Dr. Adam's words kept ringing through that it's all connected. I failed to use Google to make any sense of my issue, and so, instead of being led down a scary road of potential medical problems I could have, I decided to take a wait-and-see approach.

It felt like the pain in my left arm worsened daily, and I didn't know where else to turn. As much as I'd made up my mind to wait out the time, I had a gut feeling that something else was amiss. No matter how I tried to understand the connection of nerves, ligaments, and muscles in my body, I couldn't understand the relationship my arms had to the TMJ issue. I couldn't go to another medical doctor because if one thought the combination of symptoms I had made no sense, throwing TMJ disorder and debilitating pain in my arms into the mix would surely confuse things even more. Throughout February and March, things intensified.

The pain spread to my lower back and right arm, and when it was bad, it would be at my sides only, and when it was terrible, it felt like it was around my entire diaphragm area just under my ribs. The pain was so bad now that resting my arms against the chair back caused unbearable agony. My stomach felt as if it were squeezing the very life from me when I moved, and even though lying down gave some relief, the contact of my arms on the bed brought tears to my eyes. By this time, I could barely lift my arms to take the pressure off because they now felt heavy. The pain also spread into my left hip flexor, left hamstring, and down to my knee. Sometimes when I walked, my left leg buckled.

My neck became stiff, and I could barely turn my head from left to right. One night, while watching TV, I turned to say something to William and my neck locked up. The pain reminded me of the kind I'd had back in November. The tears flowed, and it was all I could do since I couldn't move an inch either way. I bawled and bawled, and William put the TENS machine we had purchased, on my face and shoulders. After about twenty minutes or so, I got some relief when my neck unlocked. Another seemingly random symptom. What does TMJ have to do with my neck locking up? I reminded myself what the dentist had said about connections and figured it was all the same. I had to take his word for it because there was no other explanation.

I had my last dental appointment at the end of April, and the pain was so debilitating it kept me crying in bed until I could muster the strength to shower and drive myself to the appointment. After speaking with the Patient Coordinator about not having much relief, I told her William had decided it was time to seek help yet again from the medical doctors. This time, we decided to go to a private hospital, hoping that someone there would be able to help. When the dentist came in and said he was going to remove the orthotic, I was surprised. I was so happy to get it out of my mouth that I didn't ask why he was removing it when I still had a month to go.

Dr. Adam removed the alien thing from my mouth, and it was such a relief to feel normal again, at least in my mouth. The jaw pain was not as bad as the first day I walked into his office, so there was an upside. The last words he said to me were, "Something else is wrong," referring to the pain in my sides that was so much worse since I'd started treatments with him.

My entire body felt like the pain had taken over, and 1 just wanted to get home and back into bed. I didn't bother to ask any questions until about two days later. I called the dental office and spoke with the Patient Coordinator, and asked why the dentist removed the orthotic prematurely.

She responded that, if we did go to a private hospital and they had to intubate, the orthotic would get in the way, and "they don't like that."

As much as there was improvement in my bite and jaw pain, Dr. Adam suggested that I see a physiotherapist who specialized in TMJ disorder. It was a year since I'd started having symptoms, and it didn't feel as if I was going to awaken from this nightmare. Something was happening in my body, and it was not IBS, nor was it caused by TMJ disorder. IBS doesn't cause one's arms to hurt to the point of almost losing the use of them. IBS doesn't cause one's legs to hurt and lock up while walking. IBS doesn't cause debilitating headaches, driving one to tears. Dr. Adam and I discussed the possibility that TMJ and my stitch like pain were related. He said that in his experience, if that was the issue, I should have gotten some relief with the orthotic.

The pain spread to all fingers, starting in my left thumb. Everything seemed to be worse on the left side of my body before slowly making its way to the right. The pain didn't migrate, it spread, and once it got to its destination, it didn't budge, but only got worse. In between my shoulders became stiff and painful, and I wrote in my journal that it felt like my ribs hurt and seemed to get worse with movement.

With the pain spreading to different areas of my body, the one sensation I remember is the feeling of tightening. It felt like everything on me was squeezing and tightening up until it felt painful. My arms now felt as if a hot object was brushing against my skin. My skin became sensitive to touch, and my clothes brought a whole new level of intense pain. I had to change blankets since the silk one I used became too heavy to lift during the night and caused more pain when it rested on me.

It hurt to make any grabbing motions with my fingers, and it seemed worse during the night. Walking on the treadmill became ever more challenging, since it felt as if there wasn't enough skin to cover the sole of my left foot, so it felt stretched every time I took a step. I had to keep moving as it was something my body had become so accustomed to that whenever I took a break from it, my legs would cramp up.

The pain started to affect my sleep now, as it was not easy to fall asleep while in so much pain. Then, something else started happening, which seemed even weirder. As I began to doze off, to that part of sleep where you can feel your body drop into relaxation right before actual sleep, I felt what I called 'internal tremors.' I'd already had the pounding, but this was a new sensation. The first time it happened, I thought the bed was shaking until I realized that it wasn't and that I was the one shaking, on the inside. I had no idea what this new symptom was, and I found it to be the one thing that was the most unbearable throughout my entire nightmare.

And yet another symptom! While I was asleep, for some unknown reason, I began stretching at first my legs and then my body. When I did this, it caused more pain, which woke me right out of sleep mid-stretch, only to feel my legs tightening. Since it happened quite frequently during the night, I started stretching before I went to bed. I thought that maybe my legs were tightening up because I was so used to doing more on the treadmill, compared to how much I was now able to do.

One morning in May, I woke up from a fitful night, and as my left foot hit the floor, I yelled out in pain. It felt like I had stepped on something, but when I looked, nothing was there. When I stood up, it felt like all my weight was resting on a big marble under my left foot.

My smallest toe was so swollen I could barely walk, so I had to hop around until the pain subsided. After about two weeks, I decided to seek help from a doctor, yet again because I felt the pain every time I woke up and put my foot on the floor. I went to my local walk-in clinic and saw another doctor, who ordered X-rays and blood work, as she suspected some inflammatory issues. Follow-up from her office showed that there was no fracture or broken bones, and my blood work for inflammation came back negative—the end of another road. If the doctor doesn't find an issue, the patient is left to deal with the problem; unless it got any worse, I suppose. Despite the pain, I continued to walk on my treadmill. Just as suddenly as it started, the pain subsided on its own, but the pulling sensation on the sole of my foot never went away. I was happy and could live with this symptom because it happened only randomly.

I became so desperate that I decided to try another approach. I got the idea in my head that I should try hypnosis because I presumed my subconscious knew what was happening in my body, even if my conscious mind didn't. I researched different therapists in my area who did hypnosis and gathered my information. In my search, I came across the term 'quantum healing hypnosis technique' (QHHT), and when I learned more about it, I thought it sounded more appealing since I had been on a spiritual journey, and it had a spiritual approach to healing.

Andrea was in the city, and the whole session would last six hours (maybe more) and cost $250. I asked William to take me, and of course, he was always on board and supportive of me. He took me to the session in April and bummed around the city while I spent almost seven hours with Andrea. She had a soft, calming energy about her which made me comfortable. We talked for most of the time about my experiences as a child. After she got the gist of my experience so far with my pain, she hypnotized me (or tried to anyway) and asked me under hypnosis if I knew what was causing my pain.

I'd never experienced hypnosis before, so I wasn't sure what I was supposed to feel. Under hypnosis, Andrea asked me what my medical issue was, and I waited for my voice to speak the words, but they never came. She asked a few times, but I said nothing, and I felt so disappointed because I had been sure this would yield some answers. I'd thought that, when one is under hypnosis, they don't remember the event, but I knew what was happening while it was happening, and remembered it all after. I am still not sure if she did hypnotize me because I don't know how one should feel under hypnosis. However, I appreciated the time we spent together because we talked about some things I hadn't thought about in years. I did feel some emotional relief, but the pain persisted, and so did the frustration and mental anguish.

THE CANNABIS CATASTROPHE

Things were becoming more dreadful as the days went by. Household chores were now tormenting to do. Pushing and pulling the vacuum brought a kind of pain in my arms, not only at the moment of doing it but for hours and days after. Simple trips to the grocery store were few and far between now, as I couldn't lift the bags in and out of the car. Driving was becoming a challenge, as I had decreased movement in my neck and arms. Walking around for too long made the side pains worse, and it got to the point where I just couldn't do much of anything anymore.

William insisted we had to try something different for pain, as run-of-the-mill OTC meds were not providing relief. The first time he suggested cannabis, I had visions of our trips to Jamaica, where we saw the gardeners hiding in their corners, smoking weed. Or the entrepreneurs that sold it at the shore to tourists, being careful not to step onto the sand for fear the security guards would detain them.

William said that I wouldn't have to smoke it, as the idea didn't appeal to me. I had never picked up smoking because when I was fourteen, I'd asked my mother (who smoked at the time) if I could light her cigarette. She'd said no a few times, but after I pestered her to the point of saying yes, her instructions to me were simple: "When I light it, you have to pull in really hard!"

I thought I looked so cool with the cigarette pursed between my lips and insisted I could do it because I had seen it done so many times. When she lit it, I pulled on the cigarette so hard that I think the smoke went right to my brain. It tasted awful, and it burned my entire head. Reeling from its effects, I thought to myself, *How in the heck (and why) do people smoke this crap?* It was too late now, though, as the taste of the nicotine seemed to penetrate my tongue as I tried to spit it out.

I walked away, absolutely disgusted, as Mom laughed at me. A while later, she called me and asked if I wanted to light her another cigarette. I said no thanks and left the room quickly, so as not to even entertain the possibility that she would ask again. Years later, we talked and laughed about it, and I said that it could've gone either way. What would have happened if I had liked it? She was sure, knowing her child, there was no way I would have found smoking even a little enjoyable.

William explained that we had other options, as the expression on my face must have shown my disgust at even the thought of having to inhale smoke again. And weed of all things! A friend of his, Genaro, had a cousin who provided cannabis in many different forms to people who were dealing with all kinds of medical issues, like cancer. We decided on gummies, and he suggested that we might have to try different types before finding one that worked. He started me with two different kinds of gummies. They looked tasty enough, not that I liked Gummy Bears or that sort of candy, but I was so desperate that I was willing to try it. Not knowing how I would react to it since my biggest high in life was NyQuil, we decided to be cautious, and I took only half of a 50 mg gummy. It didn't seem to have much of an effect. I didn't feel high, and it didn't ease the pain.

I was looking for relief for the pain in my sides more than anything by this point. I waited a couple of hours, and when nothing happened, I took the other half and waited in sweet anticipation for relief. Nothing happened! Our 'supplier' gave us two of this particular gummy shaped like a star to try. When nothing happened after having the first one, I took the entire second one a day later. I wanted to be sure that the first one was out of my system to prevent any adverse reaction I didn't want. I already had enough to deal with, so I didn't want to add some weed-related incident to the mix. To my surprise, I felt a bit of relief, which lasted about two days. I ran up and down the stairs with the laundry basket with no apparent pain. I hadn't felt this way in more than a year, so I basked in the relief, knowing it would wear off at some point. As much as I still didn't know what was wrong, the idea of finding some relief while it got figured out seemed possible now.

After two days, the effect of the THC (the tetrahydrocannabinol compound in weed) wore off, and I was back at square one. We had another gummy, but this one had a higher level of THC. I so wanted to take it, but I was not too fond of taking it when I was home alone. By late afternoon, the pain got so bad that I called William at work to say I was desperate and was going to try it.

I'd had a couple of experiences when pain meds made me loopy, and they were not particularly pleasurable. He instructed me to cut the gummy in half, as this one was 160 mg, to see how I would react to it, and if nothing happened in an hour, to take the other half. I followed his instructions and ate it, not relishing the taste all that much, as it tasted exactly how it smelled. I sat down and waited, thinking something's got to give. Remembering the relief I'd gotten with the one I'd had before, I had visions of getting back to some semblance of normalcy when it kicked in.

Nothing happened! The frustration got the better of me, and about forty-five minutes later, I took the other half and waited with hope. Around 5:00 p.m., William had texted to say he was leaving work, as was his routine, and knowing he would be home soon, I felt a sense of security. He got home a little after six and found me sitting quietly. I was still able to make a meal once in a while, and I'd forced myself through the pain and made us dinner. I know he'd had a long, hard week, and having to prepare dinner after that, I'm sure, was daunting.

Genaro had gone hunting and shared his spoils with us, and so I'd made curry duck. William got home, put his stuff away, washed up, kissed me, and asked if I was okay. I said, "Yep, nothing happened," and told him that I had taken the other half and was still waiting for something to happen.

He asked how long ago I'd taken it, and when I told him, he said, "You were supposed to wait an hour!"

"Yeah, but nothing was happening, so I took it," I said, almost annoyed, as he didn't seem to have understood the desperation in my voice when we'd spoken on the phone. He went upstairs to get changed, and I thought that, when he got back, we would have our regular Friday night dinner together.

He shouted from upstairs, "I'll be down soon. I have to go to the bathroom."

And I said, "Okay."

I knew things were about to get squirrelly when I busted out laughing as I looked at the TV. It was OFF. I had no control over my lips or mouth, and when the laugh blurted out, I even surprised myself. I recovered, thinking, *Well, that was weird!* And as fast as the thought evaporated, I busted out laughing again, this time trying to restrain myself without success. Then it got interesting. My heart started to beat so fast that it scared the crap out of me. I'd had this pounding-heart issue, but this was different. It raced as if I were running a sprint marathon. I was not laughing anymore. I walked about eight steps to the stairs and shouted at the top of my lungs, "HON!!!!" I heard his reply.

"Yes?"

I said, "Something is wrong! Come quick!" I wobbled back to the chair, as my legs felt like jelly now, and wondered why he was taking so long. It felt like I had called him two hours ago, and I was pissed that he didn't come as I'd asked because I convinced myself that I was having a heart attack. I wobbled my way to the kitchen, where my phone was, and texted him to say he needed to come, and right now! I couldn't see straight, but somehow I managed to send him a text.

By the time he got to me, I was hysterical, bawling, and saying I am having a heart attack. I told him, "I'm going to see Mom, I'm going to die and go see Mom!" It didn't seem to me that he was as scared as I was. As calmly as he could, he told me that "no one has ever died from taking weed," and I was not having a heart attack, and I was not going to see Mom. He said that I just needed to relax a bit.

Relax!? Are you f*cking kidding?!? I am having a f*cking heart attack, and you want me to calm down? I must note here that, up until now, I had used this type of language only on very rare occasions. Trying to persuade him of my situation was one of those occasions; I was having A F*CKING HEART ATTACK!

I then remembered my horrible experience at the hospital and begged him not to take me back there. Part of me didn't want anyone to know I had a heart attack because of weed! I believed that this was going to be how I died, and I was okay with that, I just didn't want to go back to that hospital. I started crying that I didn't want to go and pleaded with him not to take me. Finally, he was able to convince me to calm down, but only for a few moments, until the next weird sh!t started.

I sat on the floor because the sofa felt as if it was puffy and floating, and I was sure I would fall off if I sat on it. The floor seemed to be a far safer bet, as I couldn't fall off the floor. I started coughing and hacking like I was choking. My mouth got so dry that it was all I could do to muster up some saliva.

William went to get me some water, and again, it seemed like he left for a long time, so I, of course, complained that he was taking too long. I lost all concept of time, and seconds felt like hours. Even though I mentally knew it wasn't so, it sure felt like it. Trying to bridge the two thoughts proved unsuccessful and caused even more confusion in my mind. He got back with the glass of water, but when I tried to drink, I couldn't control my lips on the rim of the glass enough to drink, or my hands to hold it. He had to hold the glass to my lips as I tried to maneuver it. I felt like an infant who was learning to drink from a cup for the first time. Only half of the water made it into my mouth as I teethed the glass, trying to quench my thirst.

Then, out of nowhere, I felt like I was on a roller coaster going up fast. I must admit that it did feel good going up, and I understood at that moment why people smoke this stuff. The feeling was nothing short of euphoric! I enjoyed my ride up, even though I was not one of those people who looked forward to summer just to ride the newest, biggest ride at the amusement park. It felt liberating, and it didn't matter that I still had pain. At that moment, I was feeling something other than the pain that had plagued me for over a year. I savored the feeling, but unfortunately, I didn't think about the fact that what goes up must come down, until it happened!

At that moment, I remembered why I didn't like roller coasters. "FOR F★CK SAKE!!!!" I shouted and held onto William for dear life as the room moved toward me at warp speed. And here I thought that I would be safe on the floor! I couldn't control the speed I (or the room) moved at, and this perpetuated the feeling of the heart attack I had forgotten about when I was going up. "Here we go again!" I said. I closed my eyes in the hope of not seeing myself crash into the fireplace because either I was heading toward it or it was heading toward me. Fast!

The crazy reaction to the weed went on for what felt like hours, but it could've easily been minutes. The high wasn't as enjoyable as the first time it happened because I had the mental capacity to know what would follow. William was able to keep me calm enough that I could feel the high, which was good, and when the down came, I would wait it out and exclaim, "Here we go! It's coming again!" and hold onto him for dear life.

Then another crazy sensation! I insisted he sit with me on the floor of the TV room to keep me from 'falling.' About twenty-five feet or so to our left was another sitting room. I closed my eyes because focusing on any one spot in the room we were in, made me feel like I would crash into it. Then I felt as if I were moving from the TV room to the sitting room, but I couldn't understand how I did it so quickly. I felt as if I was in the other room, and all of a sudden, I was in the TV room again.

I had the presence of mind to know that I was not moving because I knew I was sitting in one room. But there was a constant struggle to figure out how I was doing it. Then came the philosophizing! I brought God into the mix. The light bulb became a synonym for God. Was the light the bulb emitted any less than the actual bulb itself? I answered my question, and in my opinion, it was not. And so, humans were the light, and God was the bulb. On and on I went until another 'heart attack' (or ride down the roller coaster) hit.

William contacted the person who supplied us with the gummies and told him about my reaction to it. He said that he had the antidote, but couldn't bring it, but he would send Genaro over with it. A few minutes later, Genaro showed up with the liquid, and even though I was suspect of taking yet another thing that could make this situation worse, I took a spoonful and waited.

By this time, I was on my eighth glass of water! William had to hold them because my hands and lips were still not working. He hadn't seen Genaro in a while, so they took the opportunity to catch up with each other. I was still sitting on the floor, and Genaro sat next to me on the sofa. I listened intently to him as he told William about his own experience with weed. He said he and his brother had mistakenly eaten brownies made with marijuana, and they spent six hours on the bathroom floor, high out of their skulls.

Even though I was experiencing these crazy sensations, my brain fully understood their conversation, and I kept thinking, *I can't do this for six hours.* Little did I know that six hours compared to how long it would last would have been a better case scenario.

I then felt a sense of embarrassment wash over me because I realized I might have peed myself. *Oh God, what else can possibly happen?* It was challenging to hold the thoughts I had in my head, and I said to William, "I think I peed!" and he looked at me, confused. I am not sure why I told him he needed to check to see if I peed my pants, but he was very accommodating.

After confirming I had not, I said to him, "Well, aren't you going to smell your fingers? You always smell your fingers when you touch me!"

They both busted out laughing. I was confused because I didn't think it was that funny. Under normal circumstances, I would never say such a thing to another person. It was a joke William and I had between us, as he would tease me, but saying it out loud in another's company, especially another male, was another matter.

I tried to no avail to maintain control of the words that came out of my mouth. As soon as a thought came into my head, it spilled out of my mouth without me having an opportunity to use the sense of discretion most people have, which prevents them from saying things they wouldn't usually say. For me, that ship had sailed a long time ago, and it only got worse. In my mind, I was worried Genaro would tell someone about my experience because I was so embarrassed.

His phone started ringing inside his jacket pocket, and I lunged at him from the floor to grab it because I was sure he was recording me. I thought I heard a sound coming from the laundry room and accused him of planting someone in there, and they too were recording me. He assured me no one was recording me and said that it was his wife calling because they'd had plans, and she probably wanted to know if he would make it home in time.

Feeling a bit relieved that no one was recording me, I wanted to know if I would remember this horrible night. I then asked Genaro if he remembered everything that happened in the six hours that he was high. "Yes."

I was quite happy with his response. Then he started to talk more about his experience, and before I could tell myself not to, I blurted out, "You talk too much, and it's time for you to go home now!"

I couldn't believe I was so rude to the guy who was kind enough to forego plans with his family to bring me the antidote. If this was not bad enough, almost in the same breath, I grabbed onto his leg and begged him to stay. I pleaded with him not to leave me alone with William, because he would, "f*ck me up the a$$!"

*Holy f*ck!* I thought to myself, *why in the world would I say something like that!?* It went from bad to worse, and I looked at Genaro and, in a solemn tone, said, "I hope you don't do that to your wife." He laughed and assured me that he didn't. I couldn't believe the words that were coming out of my mouth! William had never used those words, but he'd tease me because I didn't drink alcohol. After what he considered a very amusing incident when I took Ibuprofen chased with cold and flu medicine for a cold and acted funny, he kept pestering me to try some fancy alcoholic beverage, where I wouldn't taste the alcohol. Even though I was joking, having the sense to know that William would never do what I so tactlessly blurted out, I couldn't hold the thoughts in my head.

I would never make this kind of joke or speak like this with someone I had mostly casual conversations with, but I had lost all control. Even though I was well aware of what I was saying and tried not to say it, it was as if I was taken over by some drunken-sailor-alien being. It felt as though I was a separate being inside my head, trying to stop the words.

William thought it was hilarious, and he kept saying to Genaro, "And she don't swear."

I, on the other hand, was having a personal war with myself not to be so crass. The cuss words kept coming, and when I tried not to say them, I stuttered, only able to get out the "Fuh fuh fuh..." William thought it was comical and would say to me when I tried to hold back, "let the clutch out, Hon, let the clutch out."

My heart rate seemed to calm down after two more doses of the anti-dote. After a few more glasses of water, I was sure it would be over soon. I had the sensation that I had peed again, but I remembered this time that my perimenopause was in full swing, and I'd had this feeling many times before. I had stopped taking the birth control pill in November, and four months later, I still hadn't had a period. Now my rant took a very personal turn. I started to tell Genaro about all the evils of menopause: the hot flashes and vaginal dryness, how it affected our sex life, and that he should go home and have lots of sex with his wife, right now, before she hit this awful stage. I think he asked me if I would tell all of this to her on the phone if he called her. I heard the words coming out of my mouth and knew they were not appropriate, but I couldn't shut up.

While waiting for me to calm down, William invited Genaro to try some of the curry duck I'd made. We still had not eaten dinner because this episode had derailed that plan. I certainly couldn't eat at this point. I couldn't even control drinking water, how could I control eating a meal?

Genaro accepted, and I sat on the floor at the foot of the sofa, talking the whole time about who knows what. I just could not stop talking, so two conversations were happening, theirs and mine. William served Genaro the food, and since I'd never made the dish before, listened for any forthcoming compliments, as I regarded myself as an excellent cook. They didn't come, but I heard Genaro exclaim, "Oh, my God, this is hot!"

William thought it was temperature hot, but when Genaro said that, no, it was spicy hot, I then remembered that I had made the dish with a whole Scotch Bonnet pepper. William hadn't seen the pepper and served it to an unsuspecting Genaro, who ate the entire hot pepper in his first bite. I don't know how I did it, but like a cat, I pounced from the floor and onto the sofa, knelt, and leaned over the backrest to tell William about the hot pepper.

I think it was probably a reflex, but instead of spitting it out, Genaro swallowed the mouthful of food, along with the pepper. I think I remember most of what happened, but how I got off the floor and onto the sofa so quickly in my wobbly state is still a mystery to me. I'm reminded of the old cartoons with Sylvester the cat when something scared him, and he would scurry onto the ceiling and hang on with his claws.

I saw Genaro's face, as red as a cherry with beads of sweat on his forehead, and he looked like his head would explode. William was about to tell him not to drink water because it makes it worse, as he was looking in the fridge for a lime, which would help. I think his reflex was to take a huge gulp, and, of course, it did make things worse. We didn't have limes, and I thought Genaro would have a heart attack, as he wasn't used to eating such spicy food. It was quite funny to me seeing him trying to inhale air through his mouth to soothe the burn, and I couldn't stop laughing as the whole scene was so comical.

Then it hit me, the poor guy was in some severe pain, and my laughter quickly turned to wailing and apologies. My emotions were either on one end of the spectrum or the opposite end. I bawled and apologized for causing him such anguish. Poor Genaro went from suffering the burn to trying to comfort me because I became so distraught over the pain I had caused him. He assured me it was not that bad, and he was okay. I knew he wasn't, but I appreciated the thought.

After I made Genaro promise a few more times that he would never tell anyone about my experience, he said he should go home to try and salvage his plans with his family. As he and William stood by the door chitchatting some more before he left, I complained again that they were talking too much. It felt to me as if they stood there for eons, talking about nothing important, while they left me to my own devices.

I constantly talked for another two hours, and I think William got tired of me and tried to palm me off on my sister. He called, and when she answered, he put the phone on speaker and told her to talk to me. For a few minutes, I talked about nothing in particular, and she then asked if the weed helped with the pain. When I said no, she suggested I see somebody else about my condition. For some reason, I didn't like her suggestion and began to cry hysterically, and said that I didn't want to see anybody else.

By this time, William recognized the emotional polarities I was experiencing and quickly said to my sister, "Quick, say something funny." In my hysteria, I heard her make a fart noise, and she then said, "Oooooh, I farted!" On a dime, I went from a crying frenzy to outrageous laughter about her exclamation. I will say here that fart noises don't usually amuse me, but this time it served its purpose, which was to stop me from being sad.

I spent the rest of the night and the next THIRTY-SIX hours talking nonstop and trying to figure out how I got around rooms so quickly without even moving. After about nine hours, I don't think William thought it was quite as funny as when I'd first started on my rant. I expected a response from him and got upset when I didn't get one, which made me talk even more. Whenever William left the room, I yelled and asked why it was taking so long for him to return. I finally came down from my high late Sunday morning, and my jaw hurt from the constant talking. I was exhausted since I hadn't slept a wink. I would try cannabis in different forms another five times, all with varying reactions, not like the first one but close.

The second time I tried it, I had it in half a biscotti, and when I saw the ceiling move about half an hour later, with what looked like flowers and animals, I knew I was in for another ride. By the time it fully hit me, I lost all mobility in my arms and legs, and William had to help me sit up and spoon feed me because I couldn't move my arms even to lift the spoon to my mouth. I lost all mobility from the neck down, but I still felt the pain. The scary part was the actual feeling of paralysis only manifested if I didn't move. Since I couldn't move any other part of my body except my head, I shook my head and neck violently to fight off the sensation. It probably looked like I was performing some funky new-age dance move with my head.

I also couldn't focus on any one thing in the room because, when I did, whatever I focused on looked warped and ugly, so I kept moving my eyes from side to side and up and down, as it was the only way not to see the ugly images. When I looked up at the ceiling, I felt as if I would fall off it, and I couldn't close my eyes because when I did, I saw images that freaked me out. William thought that some outside force had possessed me and kept telling me to look at him. Every time I focused on his face, his facial features looked rather scary, like when something is streaming on TV, and it slows down and freezes, causing the image to look warped. Even though I knew his face was not moving around, it still looked horrible to me. I couldn't, however, explain to him why I wouldn't look at him because this time I couldn't talk.

The third time I tried cannabis, it was in the form of a jell-like substance, the dosage the size of a grain of rice, which came in a syringe. Our supplier promised that it had no THC in it so that I wouldn't get high. The pain was getting worse, and even though I'd had not-so-good experiences so far, I just wanted some relief. He said that people with cancer were getting relief with this particular one, so I thought for sure it would work for whatever was causing my pain.

I went to bed after taking it, and about an hour or so later, I felt light-headed and thought, *Here we go again!* For the rest of the night, I couldn't sleep because it felt as if my feet were running—just my feet. I felt like another cartoon character, this time trying to run but as if someone was dangling me in the air so my feet couldn't connect with the ground. Whether or not my feet were moving, I really couldn't tell. I felt like this was not my first rodeo, so I didn't panic. I just rode it out until the effects wore off a few hours later, still experiencing the pain throughout the whole ordeal.

I swore off trying to get relief from cannabis, as it seemed it was not going to work for me. I resigned myself to the fact that this was what my life had become. I had a medical issue, which was causing horrible pain, and the doctors misdiagnosed me multiple times. There was nothing I could take for the pain, and it was taking a bit more of my life every day, and there was nothing I could do. The different types of cannabis we tried were not cheap and cost more than prescription medications, yet William was determined to find something, even though I had given up hope. One day, an acquaintance asked William how I was doing, and he gave him the rundown of our experience to get pain relief with cannabis. It turned out that his wife was ill and was using cannabis with success to treat her pain. He offered us a bit to try to see if it would help.

William told me about the cannabis, and I adamantly refused to entertain the thought. Being in pain was bad enough, but being in pain and high, with all the different unpredictable reactions I'd had, was not fun. He pleaded with me to at least try it, on the chance that it would help. It was a kind offer, especially knowing how expensive this medicinal marijuana was. It was a couple of days before I gave in and said that I would try it. I still didn't want to, but I realized I could get some relief. It didn't, but the good news was there were no crazy reactions either. I just slept because I was high. They also offered Oxycodone and I tried that with no success, and it made me just as high as the weed did. I couldn't understand why other people were getting relief with these different pain meds, yet they all seemed to have the opposite reaction for me.

William also got information from them that put us in touch with the doctor who prescribed medicinal marijuana, and we thought this might just be the break we needed because a doctor would know what I needed for my pain. We got an appointment quickly, after signing up for another cannabis clinic, which had a three-month waiting period. The idea of seeing another doctor gave me hope because I thought there might be a chance this doctor could find my issue. I didn't have a good feeling after telling the doctor about the pain I was having and the diagnosis of IBS because I realized he wasn't going to tell me what might be causing my pain, as this was not his goal.

His goal was to figure out if I had a medical reason to warrant prescribing me medical marijuana. After he came to his conclusion that I did have a medical issue causing pain, we saw another doctor, who went through the different available products. William had educated himself about the various strains of cannabis, so he knew what he wanted to get. The problem was that no one knew what was causing the pain. I instinctively knew what it wasn't, so my question was, how would they know what would work if they didn't know what they were treating? I convinced myself that it was more scientific than the guy who was just selling cannabis-infused gummies and biscotti, so this was bound to work. I *so* wanted it to work!

We ordered what the doctor recommended, and I waited in anticipation the two days or so that it took to be delivered. I was having a terrible day, and when the doorbell rang, I tried to compose myself, as I had been crying for hours. When I opened the door, I must've looked visibly upset, as I saw the expression on the mail carrier's face. She asked if I was okay. I replied that I was having some pain, and it wasn't a good day today. She wished me well after I signed for the package, and I quickly opened the box, like a child on Christmas morning, in eager anticipation of receiving a toy they wanted all year.

This particular dose had only 5 percent THC, so it wasn't supposed to make me high. After the experiences I'd had, I was not too inclined to have another by myself, so I waited until William returned from work to try it. We followed the instructions, and I took it and felt some déjà vu as I waited for sweet relief, yet again. An hour or so later, I felt nothing but deep disappointment. We contacted the doctor's office the next day, and he told us to double up on the dosage, which we did, still with no relief. I remembered all the times of being so disappointed and even angry at the guy who provided the gummies because I thought he didn't know what he was doing.

After trying medically prescribed cannabis with no success yet again, I realized there was no exact science with this thing, especially when we spoke to the doctor after the double dose produced no relief. He said we might have to try several different strains before we found one that worked. Even though I knew William would've spent any amount of money to see me get some pain relief, I wondered how people who found pain relief with marijuana were able to afford it.

The quantity we bought cost $105, and with the prescribed one dose per day, I would have been able to use it ten times. I was supposed to have a double dose each day, which meant it would've lasted me a total of five days. I had been in pain now for over a year, and it boggled my mind to think about how much it would cost if it did work, because our insurance plan didn't cover medicinal marijuana. William wanted to go back to the doctor so he could suggest yet another strain or different product from another manufacturer, but I had enough of the experimenting.

I couldn't go through the same experience again. I was willing to try just about anything for the pain, but I had to draw the line. Every time I tried cannabis with no success and felt disappointment when it didn't work, it was too much to bear. Things were not getting any better, there seemed no end in sight to this nightmare, and it was difficult to experience this emotional roller coaster. Since we had some success with the first gummy I had tried, we asked our supplier if we could get more of this particular one. To our disappointment, we couldn't because the person who supplied him with this gummy, apparently went out of business. Just my luck!

PHYSIO ... ANGER?

It was April of 2018, and my first appointment with Tom, the physiotherapist, who specialized in TMJ disorder. I wasn't sure how this was going to work since 90 percent of my pain was now in my body and not just in my jaw. I did have some discomfort in my jaw, but the pain in my sides, arms, neck, and legs was more problematic. The initial paperwork asked questions about the pain, and where on the body it was, by way of a chart. I shaded in the areas, thinking this had nothing to do with the TMJ I was here for, but since they asked, I might as well answer.

Tom had quite a reputation, and as I read his accolades in the newspaper clippings on the wall, I was impressed but unsure about how he was going to help me. I didn't have an injury per se but thought I had nothing to lose by trying physiotherapy. Besides, Dr. Adam, who specialized in neuromuscular issues, had highly recommended Tom.

As I walked into Tom's office, I instantly felt a sense of ease with him. He was very personable, and we chatted for a while about my experience so far, and the misdiagnoses as far as I was concerned. He too scoffed at the IBS diagnosis, as I had no digestive issues, and said, "That's just a thing doctors say when they don't know what the issue is and they're too lazy to find out."

Then he did something that, had I not already learned about alternative healing modalities, would have made me think he was out to lunch. He asked me to hold my arms out as he touched my wrists and chest and mumbled something. I made out the words as he went through a gamut of emotions. As he said the emotion, for example, love, he pushed my arm down, and I was supposed to resist him. As he pushed down, I held my arm and was able to maintain its position. "Jealousy." Maintain. "Happy." Maintain, and so on.

All the while, I'm thinking to myself, *What does any of this have to do with my TMJ?!* But I went along for the ride. Then he said, "Anger," and pushed my arm down, only this time I couldn't maintain it like I was able to the other times. I was very aware of this, and when I heard him say it a second time, I was determined to resist when he pushed my arm down. I couldn't do it, but I couldn't make sense of any of it.

Then he asked, "Have you been through any kind of trauma recently?"

Why in the world would a physiotherapist ask me such a question? I wasn't sure what to say, and so I responded that I had TMJ disorder and had been in pain for the last year—pain that was progressively getting worse—so that was a trauma, I suppose.

He clarified: "No, like a death in the family."

I had no idea what this had to do with anything, but it would lead me down a path I never expected to start on in this kind of setting, with a physiotherapist of all people. He did some further testing of my strength and balance and also did some cranial therapy. While I was on the table, as he worked on my neck and head, I kept thinking about this supposed trauma and his very specific death in the family inquiry. My mother had transitioned just over a year before I saw him, but I considered her death more of a relief than a trauma. I explained this without too much detail, as the fifteen-minute treatment session passed very quickly. Besides, I wasn't sure what any of this had to do with my pain.

About my fourth treatment with Tom, after the usual fifteen or so minutes of cranial and other therapy, and another fifteen minutes of acupuncture, the subject of my anger came up again. I didn't consider myself an angry person by any means. And, as far as I was concerned, there was no reason to be angry. I was frustrated, very frustrated, that a year had gone by, and the pain I had did not seem to ease with any of the therapies I tried. Frustration was the emotion at the forefront, as I was frustrated with the medical doctors I had seen so far, frustrated at myself for being sick, and frustrated that my whole life was on hold because of my circumstance. I was frustrated I could get but three or four hours of unbroken sleep at night because the pounding in my chest wouldn't let me relax or woke me during the night if I even turned in the bed. I was frustrated that every time I tried to sleep, my body shook and vibrated on the inside and that no one could explain the medical reason this was happening to me. I was willing and tried everything suggested, so of course, I was frustrated.

Anger was a whole other ball game! And what did anger have to do with the pain that had started almost a year before? Tom suggested that I see a psychotherapist to explore this potential anger, as it may lead to something. The premise was that our emotions, especially long-held negative emotions, impact our physical health and well-being. It wasn't too much of a foreign concept to me, as I also believed this, but it didn't seem plausible to me that I had enough anger in my body to do this—to cause this kind of pain that no one could explain!

But, in the grander scheme of things, I certainly wasn't getting answers from anybody else, so I thought, *What the heck? What's the worst thing that could happen?* I would discover I was angry and the source of it, deal with it, and get better. I had nowhere else to turn, as I had exhausted my efforts with medical doctors so far.

I was stepping into territory that, even though I had some familiarity with, I was still very skeptical of, because I just couldn't come to terms with the likelihood that I was that angry. Things had not improved even a little. They were going downhill faster now because of my lack of sleep. It is the most disconcerting feeling to be just on the brink of sleep, just where I felt myself dropping into slumber, and right at that moment, feel my body violently shaking on the inside, along my back, and in my core. I mentioned it to Tom one day, just in passing (not that it had anything to do with what he was treating me for, but I liked his holistic approach to healing).

He used words I'd never heard before, and he explained what he thought was happening to me. After clarifying that it only happened when I was about to fall asleep, he said, "It's your parasympathetic nervous system."

My what?!

He explained that we have a sympathetic nervous system (SNS), which is responsible for our fight or flight response, and a parasympathetic nervous system (PNS), which is responsible for our rest and digest functions.

He deduced that, because I had been in pain for so long, I was virtually always 'hyper-reactive.' He explained it by using the example of stubbing your toe. He said that the pain causes a hormonal response (namely adrenaline) in the body to deal with it. He thought because I had been in pain for so long, that my body was stuck in the sympathetic state. Every time I tried to sleep, my nervous system reacted, because as the switch from being awake to going to sleep started, my body would vibrate as if to say, this is not an option, because there is still pain to deal with.

The fight or flight response is what gives us what we need to run away from or fight something that threatens our well-being. My 'threat' was the pain I had been in for so long, and my nervous system was always in ready mode, with continuous shots of adrenaline, which he thought could have resulted in my adrenals being fatigued.

He said that it was possible my adrenal glands were being overworked because of the constant pain I'd been in, and that could be responsible for the pain in my sides. When you don't understand something, and not for lack of trying, and someone explains something that seems to make an iota of sense, you sort of take it and run. There was not much else to go on except IBS, and IBS doesn't make your heart pound, give you tremors, and cause the kind of stitch like pulling sort of pain I had. I went home thinking about our conversation and turned to Google to research adrenal fatigue. I did have a lot of the symptoms, like tiredness, lethargy, brain fog, cognitive decline, and overall low energy. But not getting a full, uninterrupted night's sleep for over a year will result in all of these symptoms too.

It got to the point where I forgot things. For example, I put things in the fridge that were not supposed to be there and couldn't understand where they were until I went to the refrigerator to get something else and found them. I had very little energy to do the very scant things that filled my day. I stopped grocery shopping because I could no longer lift the bags, and doing household chores resulted in awful pain, so there wasn't much of that either. I knew things were not good one day when I drove to physiotherapy and stopped at a red light to make a left turn at an intersection. As I looked to my left, I realized I was in the wrong lane and indicated, and moved over to the left for the turning lane. As I waited for the light to turn green, cars coming from the left of me honked their horns, and one driver frantically waved his arms and shouted profanities at me. I was stunned and couldn't for the life of me get why they were all so worked up.

Eventually, when the lights turned green, I made my left turn, and went on my way, thinking about how people could be so rude. I took another route for the next two appointments with Tom, going straight on the road where other drivers had yelled at me at the intersection, instead of having to make a left turn. As I passed the lights, I got even more confused because I still couldn't understand what caused all the commotion. It was not until my third appointment that I realized I was in the wrong lane! The lane I was in was not the left turn lane but the lane for oncoming traffic! It was then I realized my cognitive skills were in serious decline because I had used this same route many times over the last nine or so years, and not once had I made this almost disastrous mistake. I was lucky traffic hadn't been coming toward me!

Of course, I was willing to explore any avenue, because now I had to self-advocate, maneuvering my way through the Internet, which in itself is a scary notion. Still, I didn't see that adrenal fatigue causes pain. I wandered onto a site with a doctor in the US, Dr. Lam, who specialized in adrenal fatigue and who offered a free telephone consultation. I made an appointment, and when the doctor called, I gave him a quick rundown of my symptoms thus far.

He was amiable on the phone and, after listening attentively to all I said, responded with, "You don't have adrenal fatigue, but your adrenals must be compromised because being in pain for that long is hard on the adrenals." He said that something else was wrong, and he didn't know what it was but that I should continue on my quest. I thought about what he said, though, about my adrenals, and tried an adrenal support supplement. However, I had to stop taking it because it made my heart pounding worse. That was the end of this road as a possible explanation, and I was back at square one.

At my next physio session, I told Tom about my conversation with the doctor and his conclusion that I did not have adrenal fatigue. He agreed with me that there was no improvement, not even a little, with his therapy and that things had gotten worse. He suggested that I start to build strength in my arms since I had stopped using them much because of the pain and feeling as if they were locked up. He recommended a resistance band, and I had to hang it on a door handle and pull it toward my chest a few times a day.

I did this exercise twice before my arms felt as if they were being hit with a blunt object. I'd never had broken bones, but I sprained my ankle once, and this pain was ten times worse. So much for building strength! My neck locked up at this point, and I could no longer turn my head from left to right. I believe Tom realized that whatever was happening with my body was beyond what he could help me with, but he thought I should pursue another avenue, stress. He suggested I go to a walk-in clinic and ask the doctor for a cortisol test.

Of course, I felt stressed! But the idea that stress was responsible for this crazy thing happening to me was unthinkable. It had been a year since I'd started losing myself to something that was slowly eating away at my very being. Or so it felt. My body and mind were both affected, and there was no one to help me. My perimenopause symptoms were in full swing now, and these just complicated things even more. Since my family doctor insisted that I was not premenopausal and could continue to take birth control pills until I was sixty-five, I certainly couldn't go back to him for help.

I went to my local walk-in clinic to get a referral to a local female gynecologist, as I thought only a woman could understand another woman's body. I knew in my heart that I was at this stage in life. Heck, there are women in their thirties who start menopause! Why in the world couldn't it be possible for a forty-nine-year-old?

I saw the male walk-in clinic doctor, and he gave me the referral and asked, "Anything else?"

I said, "Actually, yes. I've been having pains in my sides for over a year, and it feels like an awful stitch." Using the analogy of the blood pressure cuff and the squeezing sensation, so he understood, I also mentioned that, upon movement, it seemed to be worse and had spread to my arms and my legs. Without asking any other questions, he said, "It's IBS. You just need to take Metamucil and a good probiotic."

My visit lasted all of ten minutes, and he diagnosed me yet again with this ridiculous thing I knew I didn't have. I said to him, "But I don't have any digestive issues. It's just the pain. Food doesn't make it better or worse. It's just there!"

I told him about my food diary and experimenting with eliminating gluten and certain foods from my diet without success. I knew from the look he gave me that it was time to leave, and the feeling of absolute hopelessness came over me. As much as I had gone to him for a referral, I thought that since he'd asked the question, maybe (just maybe), another doctor would have another perspective. Nearly on the verge of tears, I left the clinic, feeling discounted and scared that, whatever was causing this pain in my body, it would be the end of me one day. The only questions were how much worse the situation was going to get and how long it would take. I never went to the gynecologist because my other symptoms seemed more pressing.

While I was seeing Tom, I also sought the help of the psychotherapist he suggested, to explore the anger I supposedly had. I wasn't sure what we would talk about and was a bit apprehensive about how we were even going to start a conversation. There were now two things to consider: one, the potential anger that required attention, and two, the manifested physical problem that caused so much pain.

PSYCHOLOGICAL DIS-EASE

The reason my journey took this detour into the psychological is because I'd learned about the impact emotional and mental trauma play in dis-ease in the body and wanted to explore the possibility that I had either. I met Philip at his home office for a consultation and immediately felt comfortable with him. He had a soothing, fatherly energy, and his low-toned voice and calm demeanor put me at ease instantly. We talked for about a half-hour, and I gave him a rundown of my symptoms and why Tom had suggested we speak. We made an appointment for the following week, but, in the meantime, I couldn't help but think about the likelihood of anger causing the type of physical pain I had, and, if it was responsible, why a doctor couldn't figure out the physical issue. It was an actual pain! I wasn't making it up in my head.

I do believe that if someone holds on to negative emotions for a long time, at some point in life, they will start to affect the body and manifest as physical ailments. Science has proven that thoughts have a physiological effect on the body. For instance, how many times has your mouth watered at the mere thought of some delectable food? Even more so when you are about to put it into your mouth? Even before tasting the morsel, your salivary glands spring into action. Proof enough that thoughts affect the body. But I didn't have unchecked, long-term negative emotions!

At my first session, I shared with Philip that as far as I was concerned, I had learned about the importance of dealing with anger, resentment, and forgiveness over the last ten years, after what I considered a traumatic betrayal by my brother.

After a long time being angry at him and feeling stupid for being manipulated and devastated, because our relationship was severed, I

forgave him and moved on. In my mind, I understood the power of forgiveness and moving on. I'd also learned to take responsibility for my
part in the five-year fiasco that broke my trust in my brother and ended
our relationship. I knew at the start of our business venture that something was amiss, yet I got involved anyway. Even after warnings from our
parents (as early as year one) that his intentions were different from what
he'd told me, I chose to ignore them. Five years later, my father very
sternly said to me in a phone conversation, "Don't stay another five years
and say you didn't know when we are telling you."

My reason for not heeding their warnings from the very beginning
was that I had no actual proof, as I did question my brother. I looked him
in the eye, and his response was to ask me why I was "listening to other
people." Even though I didn't have proof per se, I had something more
important: my intuition. I ignored my inner voice, which said that something wasn't right, not only because I couldn't prove otherwise but also
because it's what I wanted to believe since I was desperate for a change
in my life. I took responsibility for being complicit in his trail of lies and
manipulation, and I forgave him for his dishonesty. I didn't discuss what
had happened with anyone because I believed it was between us. More
importantly, I didn't want others around me to feel they had to choose
sides or try to figure out who was telling the truth and who wasn't.

I experienced this uncertainty for a long time, and it was not easy,
always being suspicious without hard evidence to prove those suspicions
right. For five years, I struggled with my intuition, my parents' warnings about his true intentions, and trying to figure out truth from lies. It
was exhausting! I was also a bit annoyed with our parents because, even
though they warned me consistently over the five years, I wondered if
they'd ever told him to come clean if they believed he was dishonest. I
suppose they had no proof either, but they never stopped warning me
about reading between the lines.

I said to Philip that, as much as I had forgiven my brother, I struggled
with not having a relationship with him. I thought that if you forgave
someone, you should have a relationship with them and felt terrible that
I'd cut him out of my life. I felt as though my forgiveness wasn't true
forgiveness. I'd signed up (a few years before) for TUT – *A Note from the*

Universe, a site that e-mails me daily notes 'from the Universe' (written by Mike Dooley) that seemed to come at the most appropriate time. I like his way of explaining things because of the way he incorporates humor into the lesson, letting the reader know that we shouldn't take life all that seriously.

Sometimes I had a question about something, and when I opened my e-mail, there would be a note to explain it. These notes helped give me some clarity, and I felt more at ease with my decision when I read this one:

> *When you understand that your disappointment in another's behavior or choices always stems from their immaturity, or yours, rather than their unkindness, or yours, it becomes much harder not to keep skipping through life, giddy with joy, smelling the flowers. Moreover, when you understand that with enough maturity on your end, you can always find peace in all of your relationships... Wisdom is the real deal.*[2]

I tried to focus on these positive perspectives, and they helped me cope with ending my relationship with my brother and losing almost five years with my sister, niece, and nephew, because of his continued lying.

Philip said that it seemed like I'd done a pretty good job of forgiving and moving on, but we still needed to explore other reasons I might have been angry. The issue of a traumatic event came up, as I mentioned Tom's inquiry, which had led me to him: my mother's death a little over a year earlier.

Over the next few weeks, in our psychotherapy sessions, Philip and I talked about my experiences so he could better understand this potential anger I harbored. I shared with him that my parents had a somewhat tumultuous marriage, with bouts of happiness and good times like any other (what I considered) typical family. I expressed to him that I didn't feel that Mom's death was traumatic, as over a year later, I had not shed one tear for her passing. As far as I was concerned, she'd finally found a way to leave her husband more permanently, after she'd tried and failed to leave multiple times throughout their marriage. I suspect there was a combination of reasons she kept going back: she did love him; she didn't want to be a burden on any of her children, and she didn't know how to do things differently.

I explained that four years before Mom passed, she'd tried one last time to leave her husband and moved in with William and me. She'd left the year before that too and came to live with me when I was single. When William and I met, and I told her about this new person in my life, she moved back to her home again. I'd been single more than I'd been in a relationship, so she knew that the mere idea that I'd let someone into my life meant that he had to be something special.

My parents' marital problems persisted, and a year later, sitting at their kitchen table, I asked her the following question: "If I could snap my fingers and give you anything, what would it be?" She responded that she wanted to leave her husband because she was not happy. I was skeptical about getting involved, as it would be the third time she would leave her home.

I had been in the middle of my parents' marriage from a very young age. I hadn't liked the feeling as a child, and it felt no better as an adult. The emotional toll of choosing sides made me resentful, but I felt like I didn't have much choice. Once, when I was in university, Mom left her home and went to a shelter for abused women after her husband was violent toward her. She now said she was considering that option again. She told me back then, she'd had a young child in tow, but this time around, it would just be her, so it was okay.

I couldn't bear the thought of her going to a shelter again after almost forty-five years of marriage. William and I spoke about my parents' relationship because when we met, Mom was living with me. He said to me that if my Mom ever wanted to come and live with us, he would be happy to have her. William knew that she'd gone back home when she'd found out about our new relationship because she didn't want to be in our way, and maybe felt a bit responsible for that. William is one of those men who gets livid when he hears about physical abuse against women. One time, on our after-dinner walk in our neighborhood, we met a lady who we thought was being abused by her husband. Only after a few minutes of talking to her, without even thinking about any repercussions, he told her to come to our house where she would be safe.

I wanted to make sure it was still okay with him, and so we discussed it before I made arrangements with Mom to pick her up on my next visit. I didn't know if she was serious about her decision, but there was absolutely no way I was going to let her go to a shelter again. I had nothing against shelters as they serve as a sanctuary for women like my mother, but after everything she had been through, I couldn't let her be alone.

All she took from her home were her personal belongings and moved in with William and me. I witnessed her sorrow for months as she tried to deal with anger and depression. She felt utterly powerless and worthless, because she had nothing, and as much as I wanted to help her through it, there was nothing more I could do. She tried to be happy and content, but I witnessed the same sadness I had seen throughout my childhood.

She hadn't worked for years, so she was financially dependent on us. She was devastated as phone calls came in from relatives of her husband as they offered hurtful comments about their separation. One comment made was something to the effect that her husband had said he took her back the last time only because of financial reasons. Someone told her that her husband said he had "taken her out of the gutter." With every comment, she became more and more distraught that someone she had been through so much with over the years would say these things. For months, I watched as she cried, and when she wasn't crying, she would stare off into nowhere.

One night at the dinner table, William told Mom that he loved her homemade hot sauce. He said he'd been all over the US and Canada and had never tasted hot sauce like hers and that she should bottle and sell it. She laughed and took the compliment and thought he was joking, but he told her he was serious, and if she wanted to do it, he would help her. She mentioned that years earlier, she'd thought about doing it but didn't feel she would have the support. It seemed like the perfect solution.

I could have only imagined the thoughts going through her head as I watched her mental decline. I thought that maybe this new venture would make her feel good about making a few dollars while doing something she enjoyed. She agreed that she would be willing to try, and we went through the process of getting a separate kitchen built. William knew the manager of a construction company that was building homes in our area, and we hit the jackpot when he offered us newly built countertops and cupboards, for free. The tradesmen made a mistake with the measurements, and they were going to discard the unusable pieces. We put up walls, fixed the floors, and installed the new cupboards and countertops and outfitted the kitchen with two sinks, one for washing hands and the other for washing produce. It was a tedious and sometimes frustrating process, and after it passed a government-required inspection, with my sister Kathryn's help, we got the required food license for her to operate legally.

My youngest brother designed her logo: a sexy, sassy hot pepper with long come-hither eyelashes and full luscious lips for the bottle label. I'd never seen my mother so excited about something, and it was a pleasure to be a part of it. She wasn't allowed to see the kitchen while we were in the process of getting it ready because we wanted to surprise her. After it was complete, we bought a high-powered blender, tied it with a red bow and left it on the countertop, and took her to see her new place of employment.

She was so happy that she laughed and cried at the same time. I sensed her excitement and saw her spirits lift as she scoured the telephone book, making lists of restaurants she would approach to sell her 'sassy sauce.' She was so happy that she was finally going to make her dream come true. She got started as soon as we were able to source Scotch Bonnet peppers in bulk, and she was ready to approach restaurants to begin building her client list. She worked hard at it, going to flea markets on the weekends and restaurants during the week. I wasn't working at the time, so I drove her around to her potential customers. She was successful in getting some restaurants to buy her sassy sauce and looked forward to a future more hopeful than hopeless.

She decided she would file for divorce because she needed to sever ties and get some spousal support. The day she was about to leave for her appointment with the arbitrator, she stood by the front door, just stood there, holding the door handle. I asked what was wrong, and she said she felt nauseous. I asked her why, and she said that she just felt sick to her stomach.

I couldn't imagine what she was going through and said to her, "You don't have to do this if you don't want to." She was adamant about going through with it, and I told her it was her decision, and I would support her whatever she wanted to do. She left, and my heart felt heavy for her. After so many years, it must have felt so final and like such a loss. A couple of hours later, she returned, visibly upset and drained. I asked what had happened.

"I can't do it to him," she said.

I didn't understand what she meant and reminded her that she wasn't doing anything to him, because they both admitted they were unhappy.

When Mom lived with me in 2010, when I was single, my father had called a family meeting with only three of the five children. Kathryn and I found out when one of our siblings asked if we would be there. We left work and got Mom from my place and frantically drove to get to the house in time. I am not sure what my father's intentions were for not inviting Mom, Kathryn, and me, or what would have been different if we had not been there.

When we walked into the house, my father looked shell-shocked to see us. In this very emotionally charged gathering, he expressed that he had "lived a tortured life for forty years," so we all knew he wasn't happy either. There was so much emotional pain expressed by all, but nothing came of it as far as I was concerned, because nothing changed, and the family tension continued to get worse with time. I sent my father an e-mail after we all met, but he never responded to me.

I just wanted to say thanks for meeting with us kids. I confirmed a lot of things in my mind and also came to terms with things I felt. I am also grateful that I was able to let you know that no one hates you (it seemed like you needed to know that), and I forgot to tell you that it is because of our mother that we don't. She always told us kids (Kathryn), and I, as recently as two weeks ago, "Never hate your father." Regardless of all that happened, she kept reminding us that you are still our father. If she hadn't kept hammering that into us as children, I am not sure how we would feel about you. As adults, we now know that hate, anger, and resentment just eat you up inside, so we just don't. It's a conscious choice now. I do wish that you could find happiness and not live the tormented life you say you have for so long. Mom is taking this chance to find peace, and I think you should too. You keep saying it's been forty years of torment, so I pray for the both of you that your lives become better. Maybe in your heart, you could still please your parents and finally do the things that you think Mom was preventing you from doing. I do wish you all the happiness you deserve.

All the best!

I reminded Mom that my father said he lived a tortured life for forty years, as well as her admission that she was not happy, and I said that maybe they should both take the opportunity to find some happiness. I was so wrong! Her concern was for the financial impact divorce would have on him. He told her that he couldn't afford to give her spousal support if they divorced, and if she demanded any kind of alimony, it would negatively impact him. She said that she just couldn't do it to him.

When my parents got together, my brother and I were toddlers, and my father raised us, along with the three biological children he later had with Mom. They went through rough times like any young couple with young children, and in Mom's mind, she couldn't be the reason he endured any financial hardship because of the sacrifices he had made, she said, for her and her children.

I told her it was her decision, and if that's how she felt, so be it. I knew we were on the same roller-coaster ride again, but ultimately it was her choice to make. I waited for the time when she would tell me she was going back to her husband because this was just their cycle. Not long after this meeting, I heard her talking and giggling on the phone late at night. I had seen her so unhappy for so long that her laughing again gave me hope. I prayed that this time, it would stick.

My father picked Mom up and dropped her off when they began seeing each other again, never coming into our home. There I was in the middle, again. I knew the inevitable would soon happen, and it did.

Not too long after, Mom told me that she was moving back home, and I told her that I'd meant it when I said I would support her and any decision she made because it was her life to live. Even though I knew what she'd endured over the last forty-five years, I was in no position to judge whether she divorced, separated, or reconciled with her husband.

She left when William and I were away on vacation because she said she didn't want us to be there when she left. It was her choice, so I did as she wished, and when we got back, all of her belongings were gone, along with the kitchen we'd built for her hot sauce business. I was glad that she would continue with her hot sauce venture as it had made a world of difference because she now felt some sense of self-worth.

Before we left for vacation, I told her I loved her and would always support her in whatever she needed, but that I couldn't go through this experience again. I explained to her how being in the middle was awful and uncomfortable, and that I hoped for both their sakes that they could work things out because if they didn't, I told her I would always be there for her but not to help her leave her home again.

I said it was her decision, and I respected it, but that it was too much for me emotionally, stuck in a place where I am sure my father resented and blamed me for her leaving. I knew he resented me for taking my mother in, but I didn't care, because he had no power over me. That said, I still didn't want to go through it again. Only a few months after she went back to her home, I noticed that something was wrong. I knew the signs, as I could read her like a book.

Nothing had changed, and all of his sweet words that had convinced her to reunite were fool's gold. I wasn't surprised because it was their cycle. It was just how they did things. I believe people can change, but only if it benefits them. He hadn't, according to her, and she was in the same place again. I asked her the same question that had prompted her to leave the last time: "What can I do for you?" As the words fell from my lips, I remembered my last words to her before we'd left on vacation a few months back, and I knew she did too. At that moment, she just hung her head and said nothing.

If Mom had said that she wanted to leave, I'd like to think I would've gone against what I told her and helped her, believing it was the last time, again. After all, I was also part of her cycle of leaving and going back. I didn't ask if she wanted to leave, and she didn't say she wanted to leave. She just sat there at the kitchen table and hung her head. I think she just resigned herself to living the way she was at this point, unhappy and demoralized.

I couldn't help her. After a lifetime of rescuing her, there was nothing I could do because she had given up. Her hot sauce business was not growing as it should have been because she didn't get the support she needed. One day, we sat at the kitchen table, and as we talked about her going to the flea market and such, her husband piped up and said, "She can't make any money doing that. She's just wasting her time." He said this, even though he helped her get the ingredients she needed. I saw the disillusioned and hurt look in her eyes, but she continued to pack up her umbrella and bottles of hot sauce every weekend to go to various flea markets to sell her sassy sauce.

By the following spring, I noticed something strange with Mom. She was forgetful, and it was so blatant that I expressed my concern to her. For months into the summer, she ignored me with a joke about impending old age and memory loss and assured me that her memory lapses were just part of the natural aging process. There was a time when she visited me, and I noticed she didn't have her purse. My mother always had a purse, which weighed a ton from all the coins she kept. I asked where her purse was, not so much for the money, but her driver's license and her response both alarmed me and confirmed that something was wrong.

"I don't even remember how I got here," she said. "How would I know where my purse is?" She was laughing as she said this. She had driven about twenty-eight kilometers from her home to mine, not remembering how she got there, and she was laughing about it! Her memory continued to get worse as the months went by, and no matter how I tried, I couldn't convince her something was wrong.

I finally snapped at her one day, in the summer of 2013, after numerous attempts to get her to see her doctor. I pointed my finger at her and said in the sternest, yet most respectful tone I could muster, "Listen, if something is wrong and you lose your memory, the last day you will see me is when you don't recognize me!"

I wanted her to know the seriousness of her memory loss and how concerning it was, and I didn't know it at the time, but these words were a prophecy of things to come. She finally relented and went to see her family doctor, who I didn't have much faith in, as he had a reputation of being not so smart. I always joked that he probably graduated last in his class. He supposedly told her that she was fine and should take some vitamin B12 and that she would remember everything in the morning. I wish I had gone with her to the doctor, and I don't know why I didn't, but I never really knew if he said this to her. The strange behavior and short-term memory loss continued well into the fall and winter of that year.

I called the house one day, and my father answered the phone from his office in the basement. I was surprised because he never answered the phone when I called. I heard the click of the other line, and I knew Mom had picked up the phone and was listening in on the conversation. As diplomatically as I could, I told him something was wrong with Mom and that he needed to take her to the doctor because when she'd gone on her own, nothing came of it.

He agreed with me and said he'd also noticed she was doing things out of character for her, like cooking meat on the day they fasted. My parents abstained from meat on Thursdays, and he had noticed for a while that Mom would make meals with meat on their fasting day. I said that was reason enough to take her to the doctor because, under normal circumstances, she would never do that.

Even though he expressed concern himself, he also cynically said, "So how come she remembers what day is casino day?"

I tried to quickly bring the conversation back to the issue at hand because I knew my mother well enough to know she would get angry at this statement. She didn't always agree with her husband's sense of humor and was sometimes embarrassed by the things he said and did. I knew she wouldn't appreciate his joke if it even was a joke. I knew they went to the casino quite regularly, but I didn't know if they did it on a particular day. I didn't ask because I didn't want to add fuel to the already smoldering fire I felt through the phone. We ended the conversation, agreeing that he would take Mom to the doctor. In my subsequent visit to see Mom, she told me she'd heard what he'd said on the phone, and oh, was she ever mad!

She said, "I'm not going to no blasted casino with him again!" I tried to reason with her and asked if she intended to isolate herself and not go out. I explained that it made no sense because that was pretty much her social life, outside of seeing family.

Her family doctor took her more seriously when she went with her husband and made an appointment with an organization called the Aging Well Clinic for a few months later. I thought it was ridiculous to wait that long because she seemed to be getting worse daily, but that is the nature of the beast of our health-care system. As we waited, my mother's memory got increasingly worse. I visited her regularly, and she was as unhappy as I had ever seen her. Even though her short-term memory was starting to fade, she still remembered that she was unhappy.

My relationship with my father was strained, to say the least, after Mom moved back home, but he couldn't stop me from seeing her, so I continued to visit and witnessed her mental decline weekly and monthly. Their relationship was so bad now that they slept in separate rooms, with her in the spare room downstairs. I knew she was depressed because it was so familiar to me, but there was nothing I could do to help. I tried to be there for her as much as I could, but I saw the pain in her eyes every time I visited.

On one of my visits, as we sat at the kitchen table like we usually did, she said to me, "I asked him, "Why must you treat the child like that?" She was referring to his not talking to or acknowledging me when I visited. She said that his response was to ask, "What you talking 'bout?"

I knew what she meant, but I didn't want her to worry about yet another thing, even though the way he treated me was unbearably hurtful. When there were other people at the house, he talked to me as if nothing was wrong, but when it was just the three of us, he wouldn't talk to me at all. I told her I didn't let it bother me and that she shouldn't either. I knew she was hurt by it and probably blamed herself since I was the one who had helped her leave home. As usual, when things were tense in the house, you could feel it, and every time I visited her, I felt stressed and uncomfortable.

Her appointment time finally came, and I went to the house to make sure she didn't miss it because we'd waited for so long. It was incredible that we'd had to wait months to see a specialist. I knew enough to know I shouldn't rely on her husband to take her, since they were not on speaking terms, and my mother could be as stubborn as hell. I got to the house on a cold wintry morning at eight-thirty, as her appointment was at nine, and both cars were in the driveway. I knocked on the door and waited. There was no response. I waited, and when no one answered the door, I got back in my car.

I called Kathryn and said I was at the house but didn't see any movement and was concerned. She told me I should go home, but I was determined to get Mom to her appointment. At 8:45, I knocked again. I looked through the stained glass in the top half of the door and saw my father sitting at the table, disregarding my calls. I decided I was not leaving and banged and called and banged again, getting louder each time.

Probably realizing I wasn't going away, he opened the door, turned, walked away, and sat back at the table without a word. I said good morning, as I didn't want to be disrespectful, and asked if Mom had her appointment today. He responded in the affirmative, and I asked him where she was. He said that she was in her room, so I made a beeline for the downstairs spare bedroom and banged on the locked door. After a few moments, she opened the door, her eyes wide open, as my knocking and calling had startled her.

"Mom," I said, "you have a doctor's appointment today!" She said that she didn't because it was the following day. After convincing her it was today, I told her to get dressed and that I would call and let them know we would be late. Her husband sat at the kitchen table all this time and said nothing. I called the clinic, and of course, they were used to people forgetting about their appointments and said not to worry. They would see us when we got there.

I noticed that my father didn't look well, and after telling Mom to get ready, I went out to the kitchen to find him gone. He'd gone upstairs, so I went up to his bedroom, knocked on the closed door, and opened it when I got no response. I thought he'd gone back to bed, which would be very unusual for him. He was getting changed, and I asked if he was okay and if he needed anything. Without even looking in my direction, he said that he didn't.

"Okay," I said. "We're leaving soon." In retrospect, it didn't even dawn on me that maybe he was getting changed to go to Mom's appointment. In my mind, there were no signs he would've taken her because the time had already come and gone, so I just operated on autopilot and took her.

On our way to the clinic, I couldn't help but question why her husband would let her miss this appointment. He even agreed that something wasn't quite right with Mom. Maybe he did tell her, but since she locked her door from the inside, I supposed that was the end of it. While she was being examined in another room by a nurse, I spoke with the nurse practitioner, who asked me questions about Mom's medical history and physical abuse and such. I couldn't hide anything from her, as I thought she must have had a reason for asking.

She wanted to know if Mom had suffered any trauma to her head during the times she was abused, so I explained what I had seen as a child. Then the nurse did some cognitive testing on Mom—quite simple tasks that she couldn't complete. At the end of the appointment, the nurse practitioner told me she wouldn't officially report that Mom shouldn't be driving, but she said that we should hide the keys and not let her drive.

Things went downhill from there, as her symptoms pointed to dementia. In the space of less than eight months, it was unbelievable how quickly her memory had deteriorated. The summer before, I had given her the 'clock test,' and she was able to draw the hands of the clock correctly and indicate the time I asked her to. Barely eight months later, the nurse practitioner said she shouldn't drive.

I watched my mother decline quickly, and by Christmas of 2014, she was hallucinating and couldn't hold a conversation. She repeated things said to her, but there was something I saw in her eyes. Even though she couldn't express herself or understand simple instructions at times, she seemed to know what was happening around her. She had a look in her eyes that showed she was aware of what was said to her, but there was a disconnect that didn't allow her to articulate appropriate verbal or physical responses. I learned to communicate with her differently, and we spent many hours in her bed, where she spent a lot of her day. We looked into each other's eyes as I spoke with her, and I could sense her knowing. She understood everything I said, and every time we were together, I told her how much I loved her, and asked her if she loved me, to which she would exclaim, "Yes!"

Losing Mom bit by bit was difficult, and I wanted to understand dementia, not from a medical perspective but a metaphysical one. I found out something interesting that helped me deal with her disease. Spiritually speaking, some believe that people with dementia want to pass over, but for various reasons, they sort of linger between the physical and spiritual realm. One of the reasons is that they have some apprehension about the dying experience, especially riddled with all kinds of terrifying beliefs learned through religion. I am not saying it is true because I have no proof, but on the off chance it was true, and Mom wanted to leave but was scared, I had to reassure her that it was okay. I told her I'd spoken with her mother, father, and her brothers and sisters 'on the other side.' I told her I'd asked them to be there for her when she arrived.

She would hold my hand and smile, and I knew she understood what I said. It wasn't some morbid conversation about death; it was light and funny, and we laughed. I told her she was a genius for figuring out a permanent way out of a situation she could no longer endure. I said I would miss her terribly when she was gone, and I understood and respected her decision. I reassured her that everything would be okay, and there would be no more pain or any of the horrible things she had suffered for so much of her life. I said there was nothing to worry about, and if she wanted to go, it was okay. I told her of the many near-death experiences I had read about, and peoples' recollection of feeling pure infinite, unconditional love and seeing their relatives, and the absolute joy they felt as they 'went toward the light.'

All seemed well so far, but I explained to Philip that there were things that happened in the three years before Mom passed that affected me. I was not invited to any of her doctors' appointments after I took her to the initial consultation, nor was I allowed to take her from the house to spend time with me like my other siblings did. My father never said to me that I couldn't, but I knew him well enough to know that I shouldn't ask. I didn't want to risk him saying the words, so I never asked. Sometimes, when Kathryn visited Mom, she would say she was taking her for a drive and 'sneak' her to my home for a visit. His ill-treatment didn't deter me, but it took its toll. I visited Mom once or sometimes twice a week, and on my way to the house, my entire body trembled and shook with anxiety. It was so bad that sometimes it felt like my neck would break from the tension.

I tried to believe with all my heart that my father did his best to take care of Mom, but what I saw didn't reassure me. Once, he took her to the casino and let her go to the bathroom by herself. He didn't notice when she walked out of the bathroom and out of the casino. She wandered onto a busy highway (by his description), and it was hours before some Good Samaritans found her two miles away. They stopped and asked her who she was and when they realized she had no idea who or where she was, they had called the police.

I learned of this on Mother's Day, when I went to visit because my sisters and youngest brother were at the house, and I knew it would be safe. He told the story of what had happened that day and seemed quite amused by the whole episode. I sat across the kitchen table from him, and as I listened to his musings about that day, I couldn't help but think he didn't seem to grasp the severity of the situation. Maybe he did, but I didn't understand his way of expressing it. The myriad of ways this situation could have ended was too awful even to contemplate, and I focused on the fact she was found safe. All's well that ends well.

Before Mom's dementia, she'd always complained that, when her husband left the house, he wouldn't lock the door behind him. If she locked it after he left the house, he complained about it when he returned home. It irked her so. Her insistence never convinced him to lock the door behind him, and even in her state of dementia, he continued to do this. One day she opened it and walked out of the house, and he came home to find her gone. He said that he had driven up and down the street and around the neighborhood trying to find her.

All the time, Mom had been sitting in her old car parked in the driveway. He didn't notice she was there when he got in his car to look for her. This story also seemed to be a source of amusement to him more than concern. Everybody tried to show him the seriousness of the situation, but he just laughed it off. After this incident, he started to lock the door and put a bell on it, in case she tried to open it, which she tried to do many times a day. The other thing that bothered me to no end was that, before he got Mom's long-time friend and former work colleague Shelly to look after Mom during the day when he left the house, he took her with him and left her in the car, by herself. He laughed as he told the story of her locking the car door so that he couldn't get into the vehicle. This begs the question, did he leave the keys in the ignition? If he couldn't get in the car, it meant he didn't have the keys. I didn't ask anything because I didn't want to poke at the bee's nest and be stung, but I was in total disbelief.

Dealing with his shenanigans just made losing Mom even more painful, because I was always worried that, one day, I would get the news that she got injured because of his wanton ignorance. No matter who pointed out to him that he was putting Mom in danger with the things he did, he brushed it off as nonsense, sure that nothing bad would happen. There was no way I could have said anything to him because, even though I didn't think our relationship could be any worse than it was, I didn't want to risk it. I was determined, however, not to allow him to dictate my relationship with Mom, so I endured. If there was any evidence of how he felt about me and, by extension, William, it came when he decided to take Mom to our home country, Trinidad, to visit her family (all of whom lived there) so she could visit with them one last time. We knew that, based on her quick decline, she soon wouldn't be able to travel. I was happy about his decision.

Kathryn would accompany them on this trip and asked me to go. She said that our father would leave Mom in her care after the first week, and William and I could join them for the last two weeks. Initially, I said no but gave in after her relentless badgering. I knew of his dislike for me but, when he heard that William and I would go and meet up with Mom and Kathryn after he left, he said, "If I knew they were going (to Trinidad), I would never have taken her." I almost changed my mind, but Kathryn persuaded me not to let him take my last chance to spend time with Mom, without the drama, away from me. This vacation was the last time Mom's sisters, brothers, nieces, and nephews saw her, and

I appreciated him for at least doing this for her and them. I am grateful to Kathryn for convincing me to go because I have lovely memories of being with Mom.

On another visit to see Mom at her home, I noticed a note on the fridge that she had a follow-up appointment at the Aging Well Clinic, and I asked my father if he wanted me to take her to the appointment. I didn't think he would say yes, but I asked anyway. He said no, so I helped her get dressed and left in my car. I thought I would go anyway, for moral support (as sometimes he asked my sisters to go with him to Mom's appointments). I got to the clinic before they did and couldn't understand why it was taking them so long to get there, because they were almost in the car when I left the house.

I figured I would go to the office and wait for them, and as I walked into the waiting room, I saw that they were already there. It turned out that my father had parked at the other side of the building in the spot reserved for physically challenged drivers, closer to the door. I joked with him that he moved like a ninja and that I hadn't seen when they got in. He smirked at me but did not respond, but I didn't let him get to me. He sat opposite to me and wouldn't look at me, but kept his head down and looked at his hands as he played with his fingers. I tried to make small talk but realized he wasn't interested, so I kept quiet after a while. The nurse practitioner called us into her office, and I stood up and waited for Mom and him to go ahead of me. As I went to follow them, he turned to me, waved his index finger at me, and said, "Nah, nah, you're not coming in."

I froze where I stood, in shock, and couldn't move until I heard the nurse practitioner say to me, "You have to leave."

I was only able to get out the word but before she said, very sternly, "You have to leave now. I don't want any trouble."

I begged her to let me stay in the waiting room, but she said I had to leave the office immediately. Then she whispered to me that I could come back after Mom's appointment. I left the office as I was asked to and went to a nearby mall, my insides trembling with a mixture of anger and fear. I sat in the car in absolute hysterics at how he had waved his finger at me like I was a small child doing something wrong. I needed to talk to somebody, but William was away on a training course and didn't have access to his phone during class, so I called Kathryn. When my sister didn't answer, I called a friend of hers, named Sandy, whom I also consider a dear friend. I felt as if I were losing my mind, and she talked me off the ledge until I calmed down. After about half an hour, I called the Aging Well Clinic and asked the nurse practitioner if I could see her, and she said I could come back to the office since my parents were gone.

I met with her in her office, and she apologized for making me leave. She explained that my mother's legal guardian was her husband, and if he didn't want me there, she had to abide by his wishes. I asked if there was anything regarding Mom's health that I shouldn't know about, as I was not her legal guardian, and she said no. Not much had changed with Mom, but she was not going to get better.

As we talked, in my peripheral vision, I saw someone walking just outside the window of the ground floor office, from where I sat, and instinctively looked to my left to see my father heading toward his car parked near the door. He had a small bag in his hand, and I realized he had gone to get a prescription filled while Mom waited in the car (by herself). As he headed toward the car, and my brain calculated the consequences of him seeing me in the nurse practitioner's office after their appointment, my reflexes kicked in. Before I had a chance to let her know he was right outside her window, I dove under the desk. She must have thought I'd lost my mind, and as I crouched under her desk, I heard her say, "What is going on?"

I said that my father was outside the window and he was getting in his car. I explained that if he looked in, he would have seen me because he was only about ten feet away. She let me know when they left, and I got up from under the desk. The last thing I wanted was to cause her any problems, and if he saw me in her office, who knows what his wrath would've brought?

On one of my visits, Mom hadn't showered yet, so I took her to get cleaned up. As I removed her top and took her bra off, she held her left breast up, then looked at me and then at it, and then at me again. I got sick to my stomach when I saw the marks on the top and underside of her breast, near her areola. Her eyes said something I couldn't (and didn't want to) even fathom. There were different hues of green, purple, yellow, and blue. I called my sister, who was downstairs, and Mom did the same thing when she came into the bathroom, raised her breast to show her the marks.

My sister gasped and said, "What are those? Teeth marks?!"

I said, "I have no idea," but the state of the bruises indicated that she'd had them for a while. My sister kept asking Mom what had happened, but now Mom couldn't speak and just kept looking at the bruises and both of us while keeping her breast raised. She couldn't tell us how she got hurt but was sensible enough to know she had an injury. The way she showed us by looking at us and back at her breast spoke volumes about her capacity to understand her situation. How does someone get those kinds of bruises *under* their breast!?

I wondered what had happened and about the pain she must have felt from whatever it was that gave her those bruises. We would never know how she got them not just on the top but on the underside as well. Kathryn asked my father about the obvious trauma, and he said it happened at her mammogram appointment. The times didn't match up when we did the math. I was able to go to this particular appointment because I happened to be at the house the day my sisters took her, and he wouldn't tell me in front of them that I couldn't go to the appointment. In any event, they were unable to do the mammogram because Mom kept hitting the machine and screaming bloody murder, and the technicians were concerned she would hurt herself. We heard her screams from the waiting room, and they never got her breasts on the plate to do the mammogram. Kathryn was in the room with Mom and said that they were barely able to touch her because she was in such a state of panic. Maybe she remembered the pain of having the procedure done before, or perhaps she just didn't want to do it. If anything, Mom should have had bruises on her hands from hitting the machine. There was no evidence of any bruising anywhere on her body but her breast.

The fact that Mom was nonverbal meant no one investigated how she got injured. My sister confided in an aunt about the bruises we saw on Mom's breast because she believed it was an injury that required documenting. Our aunt said, "These things have to remain in the family." What does one do at that point? I thought our aunt loved Mom and would be concerned for her safety because of how vulnerable she was. I couldn't understand this kind of love—a love that seemed to victimize the victim all over again by keeping the injury a secret. It was clear that avoiding potential shame and embarrassment trumped Mom's well-being. I wondered if she would have the same advice if it had been her mother or sister in the same situation.

I was so desperate to help Mom that I wrote a letter to the Aging Well Clinic about Mom's injuries and my concerns for her safety. I never accused my father of anything and just said that I wanted it documented that she had inexplicable injuries. I hand-delivered the letter and left my contact information. No one got back to me. Who was I to turn to at this point, if an organization called the Aging Well Clinic, which supposedly was concerned about Mom's well-being, didn't find her injuries significant enough to warrant pursuing? (If they did, I didn't know about it).

On a warm day in the summer of 2015, I returned home from visiting Mom and was spent from the usual tension that accompanied each visit. William was busy making dinner, and, as was routine with him, he listened to music very loudly and enjoyed the process. I sat in the kitchen and watched the production he always puts on when he makes a meal, trying to forget for a little while how quickly Mom seemed to be slipping away.

One of William's favorite singers is Adele, and I'd bought him her new CD a couple of weeks before, so her music blared in the background. I also enjoyed Adele's music, so I listened as he prepared the meal and sang along. The song, "Don't You Remember," came on. It was one of my favorites, and as the song started—"When will I see you again? You left with no goodbyes, not a single word was said."—I felt a lump rise in my throat. I swallowed hard in an attempt to get rid of it, and, as Adele continued in her crooning, raspy voice, I tried everything to remain composed. I told myself that it was a lover's song and found comfort for a few seconds until she mourned, "Don't you remember?… Please remember me once more."

Just then, William came into the kitchen from attending to his grill outside. He must have seen the expression on my face, and instinctively knew what was happening. Without a word, he came over and hugged me, and I lost it. I bawled and cried until I couldn't catch my breath, and I could barely get the words out through the weeping about how much I missed Mom and that I couldn't handle much more.

I knew the day would come when Mom would leave, precisely the way Adele described it, with no goodbyes, with not a single word, because she didn't speak. I felt I was losing her piece by piece, and it got to be too much, and Adele's sadness about wanting to be remembered was exactly how I felt. Losing her was one thing, but not getting to enjoy being with her without the stress made it all the more difficult to endure losing her. It was then that I realized I couldn't continue the way I was, and that soon the day would come when I would have to give her up for the sake of my well-being.

Late in 2016, her husband decided to enroll Mom to stay in a three-month program at a mental health institution. From what I understood, he said that they were going to help her learn to "communicate again." I wasn't sure exactly what that meant, but I knew there was no way she was going to be able to talk and, because of her short-term memory loss, I was sure they were not going to teach her sign language. Maybe there were other forms of communication they knew about that I didn't; after all, they were the mental health professionals. I found out about all her doctor visits from Kathryn as my father kept me out of the loop. I didn't go to the intake appointment, not only because I wasn't invited but (more importantly) also because I wanted no part of Mom being in a mental hospital. As far as I knew, she had dementia, and I wasn't aware of any new techniques to teach someone like her how to communicate.

One of the questions asked at the intake appointment pertained to physical abuse, and her husband responded that there was none. When Mom moved in with me the first time, she was having an issue with pain in her neck and required a laminectomy to deal with the problem. At that consultation, the doctor had asked the same question about physical abuse and trauma to the head. Again my father responded that there was none. He put his ego above his wife's health and didn't process that there must be a reason the doctor asked this specific question.

I couldn't ignore the irony of this and remembered his continuous warnings to us as children not to bring him shame. Yet here he was lying because it seemed as though he was ashamed about his actions, even though they were so long ago. He had to be embarrassed because why else would he tell an outright lie when asked about something the doctors deemed essential to Mom's diagnosis and care? I don't believe either doctor would have judged him, as it was not their intention. They only wanted to know about Mom's history so they could provide the best care for her.

The doctor at the mental health hospital wanted to talk to all five children, without my father present, to get more information. I assumed they probably realized they would not get the truth from him, and it seemed important enough that they wanted to know more. I didn't want any part of it, and I told William I was not interested in meeting with the doctor because I didn't believe there was anything they could do to help Mom. He insisted I go because if I didn't, and there was a way to help her, I might regret not taking the opportunity.

I gave in to his warnings about regret if I didn't go. I was not available on the day of the meeting because he and I were leaving for Jamaica, so I went to see the doctor the day before. She asked questions about Mom and the physical abuse and its frequency and asked if Mom was depressed. I told her I thought Mom had been depressed for a lot of her life, but that she was the sort of person (from what I witnessed) who made the best of it. I believed she had very low self-esteem from a lifetime of being put down and controlled. There was too much to tell, and I didn't have the time, but I remember times when Mom felt worthless because of her experiences. However, from what I saw, she took delight in small things, like when her children visited after we'd all left home to go out on our own.

She loved to cook and enjoyed sharing with anyone who visited. I think she tried to be happy, and she seemed content with her life. As far I witnessed, she didn't ask for much and was a devoted wife and mother. Because of the history of abuse, the doctor was concerned that her husband might not be the best person to be her primary caregiver because taking care of someone with dementia required a lot of patience. She asked me if I would be able to take Mom if it came down to it. I felt the room spin for a few moments, and I was at a complete loss for words. I wasn't prepared for this question because I thought they wanted to know more about Mom so they could help her communicate again. I hadn't even thought of the possibility of me taking care of Mom because of the relationship my father and I had. The doctor's question blindsided me, and I had to contemplate so many thoughts in the space of a few seconds.

In the few seconds it took for me to respond, I had visions of my mother in some facility if the doctor decided she was not safe in her husband's care. I knew she wouldn't want that. She had been a health-care aide in a retirement home for many years and had seen firsthand what kind of life it was. I couldn't bear the thought of her in a place like that.

I wondered first how I would be able to do this and second about the fact that I hadn't even discussed this subject with William. I thought about how it would affect his life. He was the one who insisted I see the doctor, and now this? I knew deep down that, if it ever came to it and we had to care for Mom in our home, he would support me because his attitude is always we'll figure something out. I was again on autopilot. What was I supposed to say? No, I don't want my mother?!

William and I were the only ones with the ability even to consider this option, and after everything she had been through her whole life, there was no way I could let her go into a facility. I grew up in a culture where our elders are taken care of by family members, especially if they're unwell. I knew she would know where she was. Now there was the possibility that she could end up in an institution where strangers would care for her.

The idea of her in a facility, spending more time than not without familiar faces around, was depressing. I left the doctor's office in complete confusion as I realized this thing was going to blow up, and I would be seen as the evil one, trying to usurp my father's authority to take control. The intended reason for going to this appointment, against my better judgment, had not materialized, and I waited for the backlash.

After my session with the doctor, I went to visit Mom. She was in the lounge area, and there were a few other patients around, some yelling and others sitting with blank looks on their faces. As I walked toward her, I noticed that she looked disheveled and unkempt, with food stains on her clothes. She saw me walking toward her, and our eyes locked for a few seconds. As I got closer to her, I saw the same sadness in her eyes that had become so familiar to me over the years. She watched me as I approached, and when I sat next to her and reached out to hold her hand, she shut her eyes tight, like a child trying to ignore an adult who was reprimanding them and turned her head away from me. I instantly felt a tightening in my stomach. My heart pounded, and my body tensed up. I tried to hold her hand, but she cupped it and kept it tight on her belly. I tried to pull her hand away to hold it, but she stiffened up so much that I couldn't. At that moment, I knew she was angry with me, and I knew she knew she was in a place she didn't want to be.

"Don't be angry at me," I said. "I didn't bring you here." She kept her eyes shut tight and refused to look at me. I knew this visit wouldn't be a long one because if Mom continued to ignore me, I couldn't endure it. Having her disregard me this way because she was angry at me made me feel a crushing kind of sadness. I tried a few more times to hold her hand, and she wouldn't let me. I knew she understood me, so I kept trying to convince her that I had nothing to do with her being there. She continued to keep her eyes shut tight, and my feelings of utter helpless-ness and hopelessness turned into something far worse: *guilt.* Guilt is one of the worst emotions I think anyone can ever feel, and I felt it sink into my bones.

All I wanted was to take her away from all of this, but I couldn't. I found the presence of mind, however, and told myself that there was nothing more I could have done for her over the years than what I'd done, whenever she'd asked for help. I couldn't add guilt to my experience and consoled myself with the thought that Mom had made her choices, and there were consequences to those choices. I empathized with her because I knew she'd made her choices based on many fears. My conscience was crystal clear because I'd always been there for her, but as things stood now, I couldn't help her—not because I didn't want to, but because I had no control and had to let it go and accept it. The staff was concerned about her because she'd stopped eating, and they said she'd practically gone on strike and wouldn't do much of what they asked of her. It was a challenge even to get her dressed.

My father showed up a while later, and Mom became her 'normal' self, even though she still totally ignored me. She opened her eyes and carried on like usual, and I knew what she was doing. Her husband brought some goodies for her; most of it unhealthy by the standards of what a person with diabetes should have. It took everything in me to not say something because this was not the time or place. So, I just watched as he gave her a drink I knew had too much sugar, and some other snacks, all in one sitting. From what I understood, the staff had quite the time trying to get her sugar levels under control with medication and was somewhat successful.

I tried making small talk with him but realized he wasn't interested, so I sat and observed. One of the nurses came by, and informally asked him questions about his ability to care for Mom. He assured her that he was more than capable. She mentioned specific safety concerns around the house, like Mom having to climb stairs, for instance, and he assured her that he had taken all measures to make the home safe for Mom.

She wanted to know if he had a support system because taking care of her was no easy task, as I am sure the staff knew firsthand. She wanted to know, for instance, if he needed a break, or if he would be able to get someone to help out if he couldn't get out of a work commitment. Before he answered, I tried to send him a silent message. In my head, I told him to *say the right thing,* as if he would somehow telepathically get my message because I knew she was looking for specific information.

He responded to her question by saying, "I don't ask anybody to do anything for me. If I can't do something myself, it just won't get done." I wondered whether he said this for my benefit or if he was just his usual ignorant self. He didn't realize this information could be useful when it came time to decide where the most appropriate place for Mom would be, where she was safe, and her well-being was the number one priority. He outright lied when asked specific questions about safety issues because he didn't make any modifications in the house to ensure Mom's safety. When she returned home, she continued to climb the stairs in her shaky, sometimes drugged-up state, because, by this time, he had moved her back into their room. I sat in absolute disgust, knowing I couldn't say one word.

When I left the facility, I felt so miserable and disheartened. Mom was not supposed to be in a place like this! However, I had to face reality, and I resigned myself to what was and that there was not a damn thing I could do to help her. I certainly was not going to get involved in a power struggle with my father because I just didn't have anything left in me.

I was included in a group chat just before the impending meeting with Mom's doctor and my siblings after I said I would be away and shared my departure date. I read the text messages back and forth, and the issue of having this meeting without our father's knowledge because "he wouldn't be happy about what we were discussing" was of grave concern. I didn't give any input. Instead, I read the messages, very amused, as they expressed their apprehension. Then the words, "So then, for the purpose of total transparency, it would be best that dad is aware that we have all been asked to come in."

I gasped at the words total transparency. As if this in itself was not laughable, it was followed by "it would be a total betrayal for him to be told by the staff that all of his kids came in to speak with his wife's primary doctor." I couldn't ignore the blatant hypocrisy! Words written by my brother, who had cheated and lied to so many people. I comforted myself with the thought that at least these words existed in his vocabulary. I wondered, though, if his attempt to be transparent and not betray our father had more to do with not wanting to anger him, rather than being honest about what this meeting would have been about: my father's history of physical abuse with Mom. I didn't respond to the messages because, as far as I was concerned, we had all failed Mom at some level when she couldn't speak for herself. I suspected that, like me, the others were just as afraid of our father's wrath and what it would mean for any further relationship with our mother. They didn't seem to grasp that it was because of his lies during the intake appointment, and not necessarily the abuse that had happened such a long time ago, that the doctor requested this meeting in the first place.

While I was in Jamaica, another group chat was started by my youngest brother, who was the quiet type and hadn't said much up until this point. When he saw Mom's regression during the two weeks she was at the institution, he decided to hatch a plan to get her out of the program.

I didn't participate in this chat either, but I couldn't stop laughing at some of the uninformed and almost idiotic things I read. I have to believe, however, that the intentions were good. However, when I read, "It is imperative that not only Mom gets out of the program but that she returns to an environment that will promote her mental health. The familiarity of her surroundings, the love of her family, the emotional care that only we as her family can provide are but just a few of the 'treatments' that Mom must have."

I had a mouthful of water, and when I read this, I laughed so hard, what I didn't spit out, went up my nose. I reminded myself that I didn't want to get angry and stressed since I was trying to escape all the drama for a while. It seemed to me too little, too late, because where was this concern by her elder son for his mother's emotional care and mental health when she needed it most, all those years ago when his words and actions hurt her? Mom felt she couldn't express herself when she did try to speak her mind (all before she developed dementia). She ultimately kept her pain and disappointment to herself because if she didn't, she knew it would cause more chaos in the family.

When Mom lived with William and me, she was deeply hurt when she heard a comment her son made that he didn't want to get involved. Honestly, I didn't want to get involved either. I knew the repercussions of helping her, but I did it anyway because it was the right thing to do, and it was what she wanted. I have learned, however, that doing the right thing is not always easy, and as difficult as it may be, we have to do it anyway. As it stood now, I had to make peace with the inevitability of Mom going back to the same environment that potentially contributed to her illness because it seemed like the lesser of two evils. I knew she was aware of her surroundings and she was not happy.

At the meeting with my siblings, Mom's doctor mentioned that I said I would be willing to take Mom if need be. When my father heard this, his response was "over my dead body." I wasn't surprised by his reaction, but I didn't think he hated me that much—so much that, if the doctor deemed it was in her best interest, the only way we could exercise the option of me taking care of Mom would be when he was dead! *Amusing,*

I thought. I suppose my father now had a valid reason to dislike me even more if the reason he did in the first place was because I'd helped Mom.

A couple of days before Christmas, my father took Mom home for the holidays, and I was glad because seeing her the way she was the day before I left for vacation was unreservedly heartbreaking. After the Christmas holidays, there was a conference call with the director of the program, one of the nurses caring for Mom, her social worker, and Mom's doctor, along with my siblings and myself. My father was not on the call because he was not able to make it, according to the social worker. The doctor spoke of my father's devotion to my mother, demonstrated by his going to see her every day, as well as calling the nursing staff multiple times a day, to the point it had become an imposition.

She mentioned some observations that showed Mom was thinking and talked about an incident where Mom, along with other people, witnessed a funny incident, and the staff observed that she was smiling in response to it. Mom's reaction demonstrated to the team that she "was still thinking inside her head but couldn't communicate." The doctor said that this behavior was in keeping with the kind of language disorder Mom had, which was a form of dementia called frontotemporal dementia, which involved language. It confirmed to me what I'd thought all along. All those times I visited and chatted with her and looked into her eyes; I just knew she understood what I said to her.

The doctor said that my father shared pictures from the festivities over the holidays and reported that she was doing well and eating. The doctor concluded that Mom going back into the program would not be in her best interest and discharged her. Her words were so deliberate and carefully chosen when she talked about my father's attempts to get Mom back home. She said that she had begun to see a pattern, and even though there was nothing wrong with it, his extremely strong advocacy spoke volumes. And would have been fairly impressive to any Consent Capacity Board, despite the history of the past (alluding to the physical abuse).

It was apparent, by the slow and measured way she spoke, that she felt caught between a rock and a hard place. She explained that her feeling as a physician, was that they were mandated to do no harm, but it didn't say she has to do good. She felt that hospitalization was becoming harmful for Mom, and she was being forced to make a decision and said, "How long do I want to carry on this battle, (referring to my father's attempts to get Mom home)? Because that's essentially what it is. It's a willful battle, and my decision is that I don't want to carry that on."

The doctor was concerned about Mom's physical and mental health if she pursued a Consent Capacity Board hearing because she didn't think she would win. Since the report coming back from the weekend Mom spent at home was that she was eating, drinking, and walking on her own, in good conscience, her doctor couldn't keep her in the program. Even though she understood all of our concerns and the fact that my father presents extremely well, as well as the few weeks it would have taken to have this hearing, she thought Mom might have begun to starve by then. She just couldn't see allowing that to happen, as medically, Mom would be much more compromised, and her psychiatric or dementia problems would go downhill much faster.

She said that she understood our concerns, and even my father did as well. He'd said that regardless of what happened in the past, he was caring for her. She said that he acknowledged that he had some culpability, but it wasn't a current one, and she would be very hard-pressed to go up against that.

But the onus was on her to present to the Consent Capacity Board. She would have to turn around and say to them, "and oh by the way (child # 5) is not at home almost every day, (child #2) lives in (another country), Sherri really doesn't have a good relationship with her father, and, in fact, they are walking on eggshells around him most of the time." She didn't have to say the words, but I understood her impossible position.

She acknowledged that everybody knew my father fed Mom unhealthy meals. Even though he denied ever leaving her home alone, I knew he did because as much as I preferred that he wasn't at home when I went to visit, Mom was left home alone and unattended. She said that though we may not like what was, we had to face reality. He was her husband and, according to the law, had every right to make decisions on her behalf. I found it interesting when she said that they, just like we, were struggling to maintain a relationship with my father for my mother's sake.

They had the same fear that my father would cut off contact with them when they wanted to follow up with Mom's case to ensure her well-being. The social worker's suggestion was for us, as a family, to be ready for Mom to (at some point) need long-term care in an institution because of the nature of her dementia. Everybody seemed to be on the same page about looking out for Mom's best interests. I thought that as much as this was an emotionally unpleasant and draining experience, maybe (just maybe) my father would change his attitude. I thought that perhaps he would pay more attention to what he fed her, and her safety, and not leave her home alone, for even just a short time.

I breathed a sigh of relief, even though it still seemed my two brothers didn't grasp the actual truth of the situation, one denying Mom was ever left home alone and the other saying he called on the phone to ask my father about Mom's meals and if he checked her blood sugar levels. He would take off to his home outside of the country after the holidays. The other was away for work most of the time, so neither of them saw what I did when I visited unannounced.

Still, I hoped something good would come of this situation, and things would change, for Mom's sake. At my next visit to see Mom, my father didn't say one word about what had transpired over the Christmas holidays. I knew how he felt about me, and there was no denying his distaste for my being in the house. I didn't care because, as much as I lived with the fear of being cut off from Mom, he had not come right out and told me he didn't want me there, so I continued to spend time with her, even with the now ramped-up tension.

With every visit, it felt like my father's anger toward me got worse, even though he said nothing to me. It was psychological warfare as far as I was concerned, and sometimes, I felt it would have been better if he came out and yelled at me for whatever transgression he thought I'd committed.

I thought things would be different because of the experience over the holidays and that she would be taken care of as everyone agreed she should be, with a healthy diet so her diabetes would be kept in check. She also wouldn't be left home alone because my father would hire her long-time co-worker and friend Shelly to stay with her when he had to be away for work. I don't know how much changed in terms of Mom's diet because her sugar levels continued to fluctuate erratically, and she needed insulin. From what I observed, she was in a cycle of eating high glycemic foods, and when her sugar levels got too high, my father gave her insulin.

On January 11, 2017, I went to spend time with Mom. As I approached her in the living room while she watched TV, I noticed she had what looked like a black eye. As soon as I realized what it was, I felt my diaphragm heave as the nauseated feeling rose in my throat. I felt my body start to tremble and tense up, and it took everything in me not to vomit. As I got closer to her, she had a look in her eyes that concerned me more than the bloodshot eyes, and her bruises did. It was a look I was so familiar with because I had seen it my whole life: shame, fear, humiliation, misery, and utter sadness. It was as if I were a child again, seeing her in pain; the closer I got to her, the more hysterical I became.

Shelly grabbed me by my arm before I got to Mom and dragged me out of the room, saying, "Pull yourself together, and don't let your mother see you like that! Your mother understands everything. Don't let her see you in such a state!"

I gathered myself and asked what had happened. Shelly said that my father had told her Mom had fallen. (Apparently three times in one night). It happened that my brother was visiting that weekend and supposedly heard the crash coming from their bedroom upstairs.

I couldn't understand how Mom fell three times yet had no other bruises on her body. Even when she was healthy, she was bruised easily from something as simple as bumping her leg on a table. I went to the bathroom with her and looked for other bruises. I also asked Shelly to check if she had any other bruises, and she confirmed that there were none. All she had was this one black eye and some bruising on her temple close to the eye. My father had put one side of the bed up against the wall, so he would have more control when Mom tried to 'escape' when he put her to bed. I assumed he was having trouble that night, getting her to go to bed, and that's when she fell three times.

I don't have to imagine the frustration of trying to get Mom to do something if she didn't want to do it because I had an experience once when I fed her, and she spat the food out—just opened her mouth and spat it all out. Even though it lasted for two seconds, I reacted with frustration in my mind. I remember getting upset because she did it twice before I realized she didn't want it and understood that she didn't know how else to express herself.

I took pictures of Mom with her black eye that day. After all, I'd made an error in not documenting her breast injury because I think I was in shock. I didn't know what I would do with these pictures since Mom couldn't say how she got her injuries. Her husband's word would be taken at face value because he was her primary caregiver, and it had been just the two of them in their bedroom that night. The image of Mom with her bloodshot eye, with hues of black, yellow, blue, and purple, haunted me, and I couldn't get rid of the image from my brain. I started to have trouble sleeping because it was all I saw when I closed my eyes, and memories I had tried desperately to forget my whole life began bubbling up inside me.

I sent a picture to Kathryn, and she spoke to our father, explained to him that if Mom hit her head as he said she did on a table, he should take her to the hospital, because she may have internal head injuries, which would only show up on imaging. All of her begging, pleading, and explanations about Mom's injury being potentially fatal fell on deaf ears, and he never got her medical attention (not that I know of anyway). Based on my father's history of violence and quick temper, and knowing how challenging it was for him to take care of Mom, the possibility of how she got her injuries made me sick inside. The only thing I can accuse my father of is being negligent in not seeking medical attention for Mom for her head injury.

The bruises on Mom's face and her bloodshot eye eventually disappeared, no questions asked. Nobody outside of the immediate family knew about this because her husband didn't take any pictures or videos to send to family, which he did quite regularly. Every time I thought about it, I got sick to my stomach. Visions of the sadness in Mom's eyes when she experienced violence and emotional abuse haunted me, and I continuously fought memories from my childhood. As much as I tried, I couldn't stop the images from appearing in my vision.

I couldn't say one word about the incident to my father because I knew he would tell me I couldn't come to the house, and I dreaded hearing those words. I already had to deal with the tension of being treated like I had done something wrong to him. Whenever I visited Mom, as I drove to their house, my body trembled, and when I turned the corner, if I saw his car, I felt my stomach flip, knowing my visit would be tense and uncomfortable. If his car wasn't in the driveway, I let out a massive sigh of relief. During my visit, however, whether I stayed twenty minutes or two hours, I flinched in agony at every noise I heard because I thought it was him returning home. It was awful, but I didn't have a choice if I wanted to spend time with Mom. I knew the day would come when she wouldn't know who I was, and I wanted to savor every moment with her, even though it caused me indescribable anxiety.

The following week, I went to see Mom, and Shelly was there, so I knew it would be a somewhat enjoyable visit because he acted as if things were normal when anybody else was around. Mom loved mangoes, and Shelly peeled one, gave it to me, and asked me to feed it to Mom. She ate most of it and pushed the bowl away to indicate she didn't want any more. I pulled the chair close to her, and we sat knees to knees. Not too long after, I heard the front door open and saw my father. My body tensed up when I heard his voice. He greeted Shelly cheerfully as usual and didn't say one word to me. Growing up, my mother always told us: "Never disrespect your father." So I said hello. After all, I was in his home and would always greet him, even if he ignored me. He sat at the kitchen table, and Mom and I were in the sunken living room three steps down. I was holding her hands in mine. Once he came home, I decided to cut my visit short. It was time for Shelly to leave, and I heard him remind her that it was almost three o'clock, and she'd better hurry; otherwise, she would miss her bus.

She replied that, since I was there to keep an eye on Mom, he could give her a ride home. The words I dreaded for three years struck me like daggers:

"I don't want her here when I'm not here!"

The sick feeling in my stomach rose into my throat, and my heart pounded in my chest. I felt light-headed and told myself, *Not here, not now* because I felt faint. I was nose to nose with Mom because I was saying my goodbyes, and, as I heard the words, we were looking into each other's eyes. I wondered if Mom had heard him too. If I heard him, how could she not have heard also? Instinctively, I knew she'd heard what he said, and I knew right away that the end of the road had arrived for me. For over three years, he hadn't answered my phone calls, and he certainly didn't call me, so there was no way to know when he was home so I could visit my mother.

Whatever transgression my father thought warranted him not wanting me to visit Mom when he was not around, is outside of my understanding, and to make an assumption would be useless. He didn't whisper to Shelly because his voice and tone were no different than when he reminded her of her bus schedule. I got the feeling he deliberately said it that way because he wouldn't have to directly tell me he didn't want me at the house. This way, I couldn't say to anyone that he told me he didn't want me there. Whatever the reason was, it wasn't the time to let him know I'd heard him because I didn't want Mom to witness any more of his hurtful words. He'd found a way to convey his message, and I received it loud and clear. I kissed Mom, told Shelly I would give her a ride to her bus, said goodbye to my father, and left. When we got in the car, I told Shelly I would take her home, as it was on my way anyway. She asked if it was okay to stop for ice cream, and I said okay.

As we stood in line at the ice-cream shop, I kept thinking about what I'd heard, still a little in denial. I couldn't hold back any longer, and I told Shelly what I thought I'd heard and asked her to confirm it. I could tell she was bothered because she wouldn't look at or answer me but kept her head down, looking at the floor. I repeated the words to her and said I just wanted to make sure I was right about what I'd heard. After some hesitation, she finally said yes and asked why he would say this. I said I was just as surprised as she was (not really) but that I think I knew the reason.

He had cameras installed inside and outside the house, and I said that he must have seen me when I took photos of Mom with her black eye. She responded, "Yeah, he asked me why you took pictures of your mother." Then she said that she had asked him, "Why shouldn't she? That's her mother!" It all made me wonder what it was he was trying so hard to hide. If Mom fell and hit her head as he said, then there was no reason to worry. I only shared the pictures with Kathryn, because I knew it would end up just like Mom's breast injuries: dead in the water.

When I dropped Shelly off, I asked her if it was okay to call her from time to time to find out how Mom was doing because I wouldn't be going back to the house. She said that, of course, I could, and her last words to me as she got out of my car were, "Don't allow your father to stop you from seeing your mother!"

I told her that he couldn't prevent me from anything, as it was my decision, and it had been a long time coming. I told her I had to save myself, as I'd run out of steam and refused to deal with his crap any longer. As far as I was concerned, I'd had enough of his passive-aggressive behavior. I spoke to Shelly on the phone twice after this, but one day when I called to get an update on Mom, Shelly's daughter answered and handed the phone to her mother. When I said hello, she abruptly hung up. I called back, and she didn't answer. I then called from another number I had not shared with her, and she again answered, but abruptly hung up when she heard my voice. A few days after my Mom's funeral, she sent me a text message and said she was sorry and asked forgiveness for any pain she had caused me. I didn't ask for an explanation, because none was needed and it was inconsequential at this point because my mother was no longer there. Instinctively, I understood what had happened without her explaining. I responded that there was nothing to forgive and that all was well.

I wrote my father a letter because I didn't want to stop going to the house without an explanation. I never told him that I heard what he'd said because my decision was more about my health and well-being than him not wanting me at the house. Maybe, if I had been able not to let the way he treated Mom bother me, I wouldn't have made this decision. It took a few weeks to write and edit the letter because I wanted to be clear but not blameful or accusatory. I went to the house after Valentine's Day to drop off the note and see Mom for what I knew would be the last time.

As usual, the twenty-minute drive was a nightmare, as I trembled and tensed my body into a frenzy. My father's car was not in the driveway, and

I felt a huge weight lift off my shoulders. I expected to find Shelly taking care of Mom because he was not at home. I knew this visit wouldn't be a long one anyway because I didn't want to risk him coming home to find me there when he wasn't there. When I walked into the house, Shelly was not there, and Mom was watching TV. I put the letter on my father's open laptop, along with his house key, and closed the radio program that was blaring. These were my last words to my father:

Hello

I just want to let you know that I won't be coming to the house after today. It may be the best thing for both of us…well for you at least since it seems that I disturb or upset you. I would have preferred to tell you this in person, but on the off chance Mom would hear and understand these words, I don't want her to be sad, even if she forgets ten minutes later. And honestly, even if I attempted to have a discussion of this type with you, we both know how that would turn out.

Before Mom stopped talking, she told me she asked you, "Why must you treat the child like that?" (meaning me)… her exact words. I tried to convince her not to let it worry her because I didn't let it bother me, but the truth is, I didn't want her to be hurt about yet another thing.

Whatever battle it is you feel you have with me, it's not really with me; it is with yourself. However, I put up with the fallout for over three years because I wanted to see my mother. Being treated worse than one would treat even a stranger is too much for me, and I am choosing to end it. My decision to give up seeing my mother was not an easy one, but I choose to because I am not going to stick around to be treated worse than I am now or for things to continue this way for another three years or God knows more. You are entitled to your feelings and beliefs about me, and I won't ask you to change your attitude toward me for my comfort. So, there is only one other option.

Mom may have believed she didn't have a choice in how she was treated, but my belief is different. I choose love and harmony. I have a broader perspective about life, and I can love my mother from anywhere; nothing can keep her from me. With her 'illness,' my relief is that at least she is not sad anymore, maybe ... and all the things that worried and hurt her, she seems to be unaware of now. I sure hope so. She managed to escape her pain in her own way. Life is funny.

One last thing: Whatever it is you blame me for, I must tell you that you give me too much credit. I didn't have the control over Mom you think I had. She did what she wanted to do. I could only go on what she told me hurt her and what her constant worry and heartache was, but she made her own choices, I just gave her the help she asked me for. When one plants corn, they shouldn't expect to get tomatoes. I am happy in the freedom my decision has given me, relief from tension, and feeling like I have too much to lose by not seeing her. I now know I have nothing to lose, so it's easy to let go. She and you are always in my thoughts and heart.

I wish for you and Mom love and whatever else you desire because I choose love. My love for you both is unconditional, but that does not mean that I have to put up with anything less than that same love. As I have told you over the last three years, if you ever need anything and I can help, you know where to find me.

Love,

Sherri

I then looked at Mom, staring at the TV. When I called her, she slowly turned her head toward me and then back to the TV. My eyes filled with tears, and I felt my stomach tighten at what I saw.

I said, "Hey, Ma," walking toward her as she slowly turned her head toward me again. She looked like she was in a daze and turned her head back again to look at the TV. She sat in an office chair and had her feet up on another chair in front of her. I don't know how long she sat in this position because she couldn't lift her legs on her own, and Shelly was not there to help her if she needed to move. I walked closer and called out again, and, as she turned to look at me, the words I said to her three summers before came back to haunt me: "The last time you see me will be when you don't recognize me!"

By the look in her eyes, I couldn't say if she knew who I was.

One of the problems I had with my father was that he gave Mom sleep aids during the day when he wanted to keep her sedated so he could leave her home alone. Then he'd complain that she kept him up all night because she wouldn't sleep. Of course, if she took sleep aids during the day and slept, it would be plain to any normal-thinking person that she would have difficulty sleeping at night. Kathryn did some research, and it was also possible she was sundowning. "Sundowning is a symptom that can show up in people who have Alzheimer's disease or other dementias. When someone becomes confused, anxious, aggressive, agitated, or restless consistently later in the day (usually late afternoon or early evening), this is called sundowning."[3]

I don't believe Mom was diagnosed with sundowning, but she protested a lot of the time because she didn't want to get into bed at night. I don't know what he'd given her that day, but if she recognized me, she didn't or couldn't express it. I was unaware of the arrangements he had with Shelly, but she was not there every time he left the house, which left Mom to her own devices. My brother's opinion in the meeting, just two months prior, that Mom was never left home alone was ignorance of the situation because the last day I saw Mom alive, she was indeed home alone. What I saw that day was not just someone who'd had a hard night and didn't sleep well. There was no expression on her face, but her tired eyes conveyed a sort of despair that I knew was slowly eating away at her.

Sometimes, when I observed how she forgot to do the smallest of tasks, it made me sad for her, and I wondered if she tried so hard to forget her pain that she forgot everything else along with it. Other than this day, whenever she saw me, she would smile, and I prayed that maybe she didn't remember all the things that caused her pain and that this was the reason for her pleasant expression. The person I saw the last day I saw

Mom was a mere shell of the vibrant woman who loved to laugh, despite feeling powerless and unhappy, and when I looked into her eyes, there was no one there.

I kissed her, told her it was the last time I would be there, and that I would see her on the other side. I reminded her again that everything would be okay, all the while trying to convince myself that everything would really be okay. I loved her so much that it hurt every fiber of my being because I knew that the next time I saw her, she would be dead. Somehow I knew the time was close. I tried to imagine my world without her, and even though I'd had three years to practice, walking away from her while she was still alive was pure agony.

I started to miss her even before I walked out the door, and it felt like my soul was crying; if a soul cries. I had to fight the tears on the drive home, and the heaviness in my chest felt like it was suffocating me. The question going around and around in my mind was whether I would feel guilty for giving her up. The answer was that she'd already found a way to deal with her life. Now I would have to find a way to deal with mine. The thought of continuing like I had been for the last few years for even another five minutes made my body tense up more.

Over the next few days, I thought about how desperate Mom must have been not to feel the pain and sorrow she'd felt for so long that she had 'chosen' to forget her whole life. She felt trapped in a life that, for whatever reason, she thought she couldn't escape, and not for lack of trying. I've never felt such grief and anguish, and thought, *Even her funeral can't be worse than this!*

I thought about the letter I'd left for my father, and part of me hoped that when he read it if there were a tiny possibility that I was wrong about how I felt he treated me, he would let me know that he was not aware I felt the way I did. I'd hoped he would see that the tension was so bad that I was willing to give up Mom, and he would put aside whatever grouse he had with me because we all had limited time with her. I didn't expect him to do a complete one-eighty, but maybe we could've come to an understanding that would allow me to comfortably spend time with her, like my other siblings did, taking her to their homes sometimes for days or even a week. I waited for the phone to ring and for him to be a father, and call a truce so that we could be together in the same room without the tension.

His phone call never materialized, and I decided I had made the right choice by not going back to the house. I think I know my father well enough to know if this ever came up in a conversation, he would say it was my choice to give up my mother; he would be right. It was the only choice I felt I had for the sake of my mental health, and I don't regret my decision; I just regret feeling like I had to do it to save myself.

There were a few things that happened in the years leading up to Mom's dementia that added to her already painful life experience. She took her children's actions and behavior very personally. It was different from my father's feeling of being shamed by our actions, as he was more concerned about his reputation. Mom, on the other hand, felt a responsibility and took the blame, so to speak, as though she was the one who did something wrong. As much as I tried to convince her that everyone had to live their own lives, she harbored and internalized her pain. About her elder son's actions, she wrote me an e-mail about her feelings and said, "I am so hurt and disappointed, not to mention ashamed… The question going round and round in my head is what have I done to my children that was so terrible that they must hurt me so bad in order to find their happiness?"

She took it as a personal parenting flaw as a mother that she wasn't successful in teaching essential personality traits, like honesty and integrity. I kept reminding her of an adage I'd heard growing up that you make the children, but you don't make their minds. I understood that it was not necessarily the choices made, but how things were done, specifically regarding her elder son, whom she respected.

I believe parents have different relationships with each of their children because each child has their unique characteristics. Mom and I had a special connection because I was her eldest, but I knew she also had a special bond with my brother because he was her firstborn son. She said she "lost all respect for him" because of his lies, deceit, and manipulation to get his happiness at the expense of others. To add insult to injury, when she tried to express her disappointment and pain to him, she felt she was shut down and disrespected, and she never got over it. According to her, he answered her with total disregard. She felt so hurt and said, "I love him; he is my son, but that day he lost me. This has just turned the knife to the extreme."

Mom just wouldn't let it go, no matter how much I tried to tell her she had to. I was more concerned about her mental health than standing up for my brother. She talked about it for years after, until she started to turn off her light switch. She never got over him discounting her feelings, as if she didn't matter.

What made it all the more unbearable was that she had to engage with him, with her feelings bottled up, because expressing it would have caused more problems in the family. She couldn't avoid family gatherings because to say she wouldn't go only caused more tension, so she just went along while feeling powerless, and interestingly, voiceless.

Before she became nonverbal, one day, when she was home alone, she looked out the window to see relatives in the driveway who'd made an unannounced visit. She quickly ran into the crawl space in the basement and stayed there for hours, so she didn't have to deal with them. Of course, her husband had left the front door open, so they invited themselves in and waited for someone's arrival. It wasn't too long after they got there that he came home and was none the wiser that Mom was hiding in the basement, just to avoid socializing with family.

She told me this after the fact, and I told her how insane it was. Even though it was summer, the crawl space was dark, musty, cold, and filled with stuff gathered over thirty years. To think that she sat there for that long was alarming, but I suppose it was her way of dealing with a situation she felt she couldn't deal with any other way. I don't know where her husband thought she was because she was still driving at the time, and her car was in the driveway. I admired how my mother was able to have such a bubbly personality when she was with family and friends even while feeling extremely unhappy on the inside, hiding her hurt and pain. Unfortunately (or fortunately), it's not a trait I inherited from her.

I, too, had my moments with Mom over the years. For example, when I was sixteen and fighting for some semblance of independence, I wanted to attend a classmate's gathering at his home. It was a traditional Hindu prayer event, and she wouldn't give me a reason why I couldn't go, except "because I said so," which never sat well with me. We argued back and forth for a bit until the words "I don't know why you didn't flush me down the toilet" fell out of my mouth before my brain could register the pain this would cause her.

Mom was nineteen when she became pregnant with me, and I knew the trauma of her young life. Saying those awful words, I am sure, hurt her to the core of her being. By the time I realized the hurtful words I angrily yelled at her, it was too late, and I knew the impending repercussions as she lunged at me. I ran as fast as I could to my father, who was sitting in his recliner. I stood in front of him and said, help me, and he responded, "Don't get me involved in your thing."

It was apparent I wasn't going to be rescued, and as she came toward me, I ran into a bedroom where there were two beds. I jumped from one to the other and played cat and mouse with her until she was too tired and gave up. I joked with her many years later that the only reason I was alive today is because I was able to outrun her. It was on this day I made a conscious decision that I would never disrespect her again and that one day, I would grow up and do what I wanted. I could never take back those horrible words and the pain I saw in her eyes, and I made a promise to never say hurtful words to her no matter how angry I was. We had our disagreements about all sorts of things over the years, from me meeting my biological father (which she adamantly opposed) to discussions about race and my relationships, and other touchy subjects on which we didn't agree. Still, I was always careful not to use words to hurt her.

The straw that broke the camel's back and that contributed to her depression and rapid mental deterioration, however, was her suspicion that her husband had cheated on her. She learned that he had reconnected with an old girlfriend after her husband died. She became obsessed with this and was so hurt and angry, and it was the reason she moved in with me the first time before William and I got together. She was devastated, and as her memory started its decline, her obsession got worse. She told me she'd heard him through the vents at all hours of the night, talking to the woman.

I told Mom that I didn't think there was anything to worry about, not because I believed there was no reason for her worry but because I saw what it did to her. I understood that she might not have necessarily thought her husband was having a physical affair, but that he kept in touch with this person was reason enough for her to be angry and hurt.

She said that he called the woman from his office, and I asked her how she knew that because she wasn't at the office. She told me she had gone to the office with him and had seen the woman's phone number on the phone bills. As her mental state got worse, she told me that once she'd hit redial on the home phone to see if her husband called the lady. She said she heard the number 977-997-7799, and that she knew it was the lady's number. I knew those numbers were actually from when the voice mail was accessed, and as the messages were played and deleted or saved, and not an actual phone number. But Mom's sense of logic was already slipping, so she insisted it was the woman's phone number.

To prove her wrong, I asked her to get me the phone bill so I could show her that she fretted over nothing. When she showed me the long-distance numbers on the bill, I explained that those were her sister's phone numbers, pointing at it while reciting the numbers. I saw other long-distance numbers I didn't recognize and quickly folded the bill before she could see them and ask whose they were.

I fought a losing battle, trying to convince Mom she was wrong, and even when she lost most of her vocabulary, the first question out of her mouth, if she talked to her husband on the phone, was whether or not he was talking to the woman. I knew my father kept in touch with this lady because on one of my visits to see Mom, I saw a local cookbook on the coffee table, and it piqued my interest. A few weeks before, he had gone on vacation, leaving Mom in Kathryn's care (even though I lived closer), and the book had appeared at the house after his return.

I thumbed through the book, and when I got to the back, I saw a photo of the lady and a message that she had inscribed. I was thankful Mom couldn't read at this point, as this would've been more than enough to prove her suspicions, and I am sure it would have made things worse. Even though I wasn't successful in convincing her there was nothing to worry about, I understand that her pain stemmed from the mere act of him keeping in touch with this person against her wishes, even though she'd told him how she felt.

I can't imagine how discounted and worthless she must have felt because even though she'd expressed her feelings and obvious insecurity, these were not validated as he continued his friendship with the lady. I'm not saying Mom was right or wrong to be angry, but it was just another thing that she held on to and allowed to eat her up inside. She spoke about it until she became nonverbal and couldn't talk about it anymore. I often prayed that, if she didn't talk about it, maybe she forgot the pain it caused her. How can one be sure? According to her doctor at the mental hospital, Mom was thinking inside her head. Everybody who interacted with her said the same thing, that she was aware of everything around her, even though she was unable to express herself verbally.

It was a Sunday morning, March 12, 2017, when I got the call from my youngest brother. I was in the shower and heard the phone ring twice. When I got out, I saw that I had two missed calls from him. I knew something was wrong because he rarely kept in touch, and him calling twice in the space of ten minutes meant something was amiss. I called him back, and he answered.

"Come now; something is wrong with Mom!" I told him I'd just gotten out of the shower and would leave as soon as I dried my hair.

He was adamant. "No, you have to come now!"

It was a cold morning, so I put a hat on to keep my wet hair from freezing and yelled out to William that we were going to Mom's because something was wrong. As we drove to the house, a sense of relief and peace suddenly washed over me because I knew she was gone. It had been barely three weeks since I'd last seen her.

When we got to the house, the police were there. That was normal, I supposed, as I'd never had an experience like this. My father was sitting at the kitchen table, relaying the news to some relatives on the phone. As I walked toward him, I noticed that he was crying, and I felt anger rise in me. When he had the opportunity to treat Mom with some respect, he hadn't, so why the tears now? I quickly reminded myself that, despite their history together, he too had lost someone—his wife of over forty years—and told myself that I should have some compassion for him.

He didn't look in my direction, and I remembered that he didn't want me there (when he wasn't there), but I knew it was the last time I would be in this house. I knew he wouldn't mistreat me when other people were around, so I felt safe. I asked the female police officer where Mom was, and she indicated that she was upstairs in the bedroom. I made a beeline for the stairs, but she cut me off and said I couldn't go upstairs. She asked who I was, and I told her I was Mom's eldest daughter. The police officer explained that sometimes seeing a deceased parent is too traumatic, and she advised against it. I assured her that I was quite capable of seeing my dead mother, and I would be okay. She hesitantly let me go and said that they were waiting for the coroner to pronounce Mom.

I said, "Okay, I will be fine. I will wait upstairs."

Mom was lying on the floor with the tube in her mouth from when paramedics had attempted to resuscitate her. I looked at her and immediately felt like a hundred pounds were lifted off my shoulders. I felt a sense of relief and joy and thought I must be going crazy because those emotions were not normal. I had been preparing myself for this for so long that it seemed like the next logical step, but feeling joy didn't seem appropriate.

I sat beside her and kissed her, and her skin was cold as she had passed in her sleep. The windows were open, and the cold winter breeze filled the room. I tried to take the tube out of her mouth, but I didn't know the technique to remove it. I rested my head on her tummy for what felt like more than two hours and talked to my dead mother. We (or I) laughed as I asked who was there to greet her, calling the names of her deceased relatives and my biological father, who I knew she didn't like very much. I told her I knew she was okay now and that there was no more pain where she was.

As I rested on Mom's tummy, I heard someone coming up the stairs and put my solemn face on. When I looked up, I saw my father. I looked at him for two seconds before lying back on Mom, wondering what was going through his head. Did he think about the past and how he had treated her? Did he have any regrets? Did he wish he'd done things differently? Was he relieved he didn't have to take care of her anymore because he'd told Shelly she gave him a lot of trouble? I wasn't angry with him anymore for how difficult he'd made it for me to spend time with Mom in her last days. I kept reminding myself that he too had suffered a loss, and even though I prepared myself for this day, it seemed he didn't because he said her passing surprised him.

I noticed that he looked tired, and I did feel for him. I reminded myself again that compassion was the most appropriate response in that moment. Everybody, myself included, was aware of the toll a caregiver experiences in situations like this. I'd heard a comment made by someone named Fiona—who liked to give her unsolicited opinion without all the necessary information—that my father would probably die before Mom because of the stress she caused him. I'm not saying taking care of Mom didn't have its strains, and Kathryn and I had conversations many times about our concern for his health. However, we found it difficult to have much empathy for him because a lot of his stress was self-inflicted.

There were a myriad of ways he could have reduced some of the challenges that came with taking care of Mom. He could have educated himself about both her diabetes and dementia, as well as accept (or at the very least consider) the advice of those who did spend time researching Mom's issues to understand them better. Maybe he did research her condition, I don't know, but his actions didn't show that he was knowledgeable about the complications that accompanied Mom's medical conditions. He could have tried to create a calmer environment for her when she became nonverbal, and he could have shown more empathy by not teasing her to the point where she screamed until her voice became hoarse. Also, he could not have shut me out because I was not working and had more time than anybody else to help out. Instead, his disdain for me and his pigheadedness got in the way. He chose to cut off his nose to spite his face, but, in the end, I concluded that it was his prerogative to do so.

William always says to me, life is about choice, and from what I observed, my father chose to do things the difficult way. I don't know how long he stood there, watching me with my head on Mom's tummy. My father's brother and his wife came up to the room where Mom and I were, and my uncle rustled my hair like one would do to a child, and I understood he was relaying his sympathy. They didn't stay very long, and as soon as they left, I continued my conversation with Mom, telling her how happy I was that she was now okay, and there was no more pain where she was, whether physical or emotional.

I kissed her hands and felt a sort of euphoria. However, I kept questioning my sanity because I was not supposed to feel like this. I comforted myself with the thought that I must not be crazy, because crazy people don't question whether they are insane. (I use the term loosely and not in a derogatory way; it was just what was going through my head at that moment). I still felt like the usual protocol when one's mother dies is to feel sadness, and maybe cry, especially if they were as close as Mom and I were. I had no tears, even when I thought I should perhaps try to cry because I certainly didn't feel sad. Even though her skin was cold, I wanted to remember the sensation of her touch one last time. I thanked her for choosing her demise because it gave me time to deal with her leaving. (I say leaving because the word death seems so final, and it's not how I felt now that she was no longer here.)

I told Mom that the three years she was ill had given me time to get used to the feeling of her not being around because, even though she was there in body, it was like she was not there. Our relationship changed because of the dementia, and it was easier to handle her leaving because I'd had three years to say goodbye gradually. If she had suddenly left, I think it would have been more difficult to deal with not having her around.

I told her that I would not be attending her funeral because we had talked about her wishes, and I knew her husband would do the opposite of everything she wanted. I said I wouldn't be a witness to his dog and pony show. I told her it was more important to me how we treat each other while we are alive, not when we are no longer in physical form. I knew it would be a spectacular show, and I wanted no part of it. I said that this was my last goodbye, and I hoped I wouldn't have regrets about the decision I'd made.

When the coroner showed up, I left the room and spoke to my youngest brother, who was probably still in a state of shock as he had been the one who'd tried to resuscitate Mom when they realized something was wrong. He was visibly upset and sad, and I am sure he was in pain, as he is the baby of the family. He too expressed surprise Mom had left because he said that she was fine the night before and had shown no signs of being in distress. He'd played the guitar for her, and she'd enjoyed their time together as he visited that weekend.

None of it mattered to me, as I knew in my heart of hearts that Mom was in a much better place. While I was there, Shelly came by, and she too expressed surprise; she had been at the house the night before and said everything seemed well with Mom. She said that Mom had pizza for dinner, and "your dad even gave her sugar water and insulin before she went to bed."

I stopped dead in my tracks and was utterly astounded by this statement! Before I could ask for clarification, I realized they were bringing Mom down the stairs. I didn't want to see them take her out of the house in a body bag, as the image would haunt me forever. I already had too many images that I was trying not to think about to add this one to my memory bank. I didn't have time to ask any other questions regarding this startling information because I wanted to make a speedy exit. On the way home, I told William what Shelly had said, and he was shocked. We contemplated why someone would give a diabetic sugar water when their sugar level was already too high. Mom's sugar level was so high she was already on insulin, so as far as I understood, sugar water would make the situation worse.

Mom had been diagnosed with diabetes when she was fifty, and in all the years of her dealing with this disease, as far I knew, her sugar levels were never as low as to require a sugar-water concoction. I didn't pursue a potential reason, even though it bothered me and will forever remain a mystery, partly because I don't want to know, and Mom isn't here to say anything. The coroner said that Mom's heart gave up, and she died in her sleep. Even though there was no autopsy to ascertain the cause of death, her death certificate states she died of myocardial infarction and that she'd had coronary artery disease for ten years.

The first time I heard anything about her having CAD for this long was when Kathryn told me, two years after Mom left. I'd never heard about Mom having this condition in all the time she was unwell or even before. As far as we knew, her heart was surprisingly healthy, even though she had diabetes. When I heard that her heart gave up, knowing she had no heart issues her whole life, I wondered if it was because it was so broken and sad. It didn't matter at this point because, as far as I was concerned, she was her true self once again: pure, divine consciousness.

My father arranged the cremation for the following Thursday. Although I made the decision not to be a part of it, Kathryn kept me abreast of the planning. At the back of my mind, I still questioned my decision not to attend because I didn't want guilt or regret added to the unpleasant emotions I already had on my plate. Kathryn called me on Tuesday night and said that she and two aunts were going to get Mom ready for the viewing on Wednesday and asked if I wanted to be a part of it. I told her I didn't think so because I was afraid this would be my last memory of Mom, and I already had one of her on the floor of her bedroom with the tube in her mouth. This was only partly the reason for my hesitation as what I didn't want, was the feeling of her cold embalmed skin in a funeral home to be the last thing I felt. When I was a young teen, my mother took me with her to help get an old aunt of ours who'd passed ready for her funeral, and it freaked me out how different the embalmed body felt to the touch.

I'd spent the last three years holding and touching Mom because that's the memory I wanted to keep of her when she was no longer around. Kathryn said that I shouldn't make a decision right away and should sleep on it and call her the next morning. If I decided to go, she wanted me to bring a dozen white carnations.

As we got ready for bed, William insisted on helping me relieve some stress because all the anxiety and trauma since Mom left our home to move back to her home, was now all over. I was a bit hesitant at first because it felt weird; I wondered if Mom was in the room. William joked that if she were, she would probably be jealous while cheering me on. Knowing my Mom, I agreed with him, and, by the time I was ready for bed, I was relaxed and content. As I basked in the afterglow, I thought I would have a chat with Mom and whispered to her that if she could hear me, I needed to ask her something very important.

I said that I'd already made up my mind not to attend her funeral but feared the regret if I didn't. I also told her I was of two minds about going the next morning to help get her dressed. I felt like a weight was lifted off me as I imagined Mom finally being at peace wherever she was. I no longer saw the horrible images of her with her injuries over the last few months, and I quickly fell off into a deep slumber.

I was awakened by William's moving about. It was morning and time for him to get ready for work. I immediately searched through my memory for a dream I may have had during the night, but alas, there was nothing. A bit disappointed, I dozed back to sleep as I listened to William head downstairs to begin his morning routine. I heard him come back up a while later and get into the shower.

I fell asleep again and had the most amazing and beautiful experience, incomparable to any experience I had with Mom when she was alive. I suddenly felt my mother's presence and heard her unique laugh! I don't know what she was laughing at, but I started laughing too! Her distinctive laugh was one everybody knew, and there was no question in my mind that it was her. Then I suddenly joined her where she was, hovering in absolute nothingness while the sweetest music I'd ever heard played in the background.

I questioned myself, wondering if I recognized what musical instruments they were, as it was the most enchanting melody I had ever heard. I couldn't figure out what instruments played, but what I did know was that I'd never heard music like this before. *And where were we?* There was no scenario or familiar surroundings like one may remember having in a dream. Mom and I just hovered, holding each other's hands. I didn't see us in physical form either. It was as if I was visualizing the scenario, so it was not like a dream where you see actual images. The best way I can describe the place we were in is, it's what you see when you close your eyes in a dark room—just nothing. No beginning and no end. No color or texture. We were both holding each other in this mid-nothingness. She laughed and laughed, and we 'jumped' up and down like we'd just won a big prize. The feeling of joy I had, deep down in my solar plexus, felt like pure bliss, a feeling I'd never felt before.

I felt such happiness, peace, and love all at the same time. I could hear Mom's voice clear as day as if she were right in the room with me. I didn't speak words, but as if by telepathy, she heard my thought: *I don't want to go to your funeral.*

Just as quickly as I had the thought, I heard her say, "It's glorious for all of us!" and we jumped up and down in mid-air, holding hands and laughing while the beautiful music played. I told myself that I had to remember what she said, and it was easy because it rhymed. I was having a conversation with myself while this was happening, and at the same time questioning what it meant. Then somehow, in that moment, I knew it was okay not to go to her funeral. I felt relieved and knew it was Mom because there was no other way to explain this experience.

As this understanding sunk in, my thought quickly shifted to my second question: helping to get her ready for her viewing. Suddenly, she moved out of the nothingness we danced in, to the side of the bed next to me. I was then facing her, and I questioned myself how she even got there because I wasn't aware that she'd moved. I knew I was facing the other direction; how did I turn without even knowing?

I then felt a pair of hands hold mine again. It felt so real that, for a few seconds, I thought it was William. By now, he should be ready to leave for work and would have come to kiss me goodbye. I tried to figure out what was happening because it didn't smell like William when I sniffed the air for the mild smell of his cologne, which usually lingered for hours after he left for work. I couldn't smell him and directed my attention to the hands holding mine, trying to figure out in my mind whose hands they were. I thought to myself again that it must be William holding my hands because they felt so familiar. After a few seconds, I realized they weren't William's hands after all. Mom was holding my hands! The many times she and I spent time in her bed, when I held her hands, felt nothing like this!

The profound feeling of joy felt as if it came straight from her as she held my hands. Then, as if through sheer thought transference, she felt my confusion and cupped my face. Again, I just knew my worry was in vain, and what I would remember was this moment right here, right now, where I felt the warmth of her hands on my cheeks.

As I thought, *Okay, I get it*, it was all over. Mom was gone, but it felt as though my heart would explode with joy. The feeling in my solar plexus felt as if I were going down fast in a roller coaster. Just at that moment, I felt William coming toward me as I usually do, even if I am deep in sleep.

By the time he got to me, I had blurted out, "She came! She came!" He, of course, was startled by my outburst, but after we spoke about it, he said I was laughing in my sleep as he'd approached to kiss me goodbye.

Mom had come and answered both my questions, so the next morning, I bought twelve white carnations to make a sort of necklace for her (called a mala in Hindu tradition), and headed to the funeral home. I didn't know my father was coming to the funeral home, but Kathryn gave me a heads-up when she saw his vehicle. I took my flowers and went upstairs to another room because I didn't want to be in his presence. I knew he would talk to me as if the last nine years hadn't happened.

As I sat on the stairs making the mala, I thought about how ridiculous it was and decided I wasn't going to hide from him any longer. I gathered up my carnations, needle, and thread and headed back down the stairs to the room where Mom was on the cold, stainless-steel table.

He came into the room and greeted my two aunts and sisters with the usual hugs and kisses, and then he headed in my direction. When I saw him coming, I thought to myself, *You better not*, and when he did, I felt the words, are you for real right now, about to come out of my mouth but stopped myself, hearing my mother's words again: "Never disrespect your father."

I kept quiet and allowed him to kiss and greet me because, based on a lifetime of experience of Mom stopping me when I tried to express my disgust at his behavior, I was sure she would open her eyes and give me 'the look.' Even as an adult, I knew when I stepped out of bounds with Mom when she gave me that look, the one that needed no words to convey her message that I was on the verge of being disrespectful.

My father kissed me as if we had spoken the day before, and I allowed him to, partly because I was very familiar with his public persona. I also knew this would be the last time that I would be a party to one of his hypocritical displays. I watched as he performed the rituals for the physical body, using water he'd brought that he acquired from someone's visit to the Ganges River in India. It was important to him to do the things necessary to ensure Mom's soul went to its rightful place. Observing him confirmed to me that I'd made the right decision about not going to Mom's cremation, where there would be more of these sacraments performed. Even more would be done six months and a year after Mom left, again in efforts to help her soul on its journey.

It was difficult for me to truly understand how one could treat another person with such disrespect and, at times, contempt, when they were alive and, when the person dies, go to such great lengths to respect the soul. To carry out these religious formalities to ensure the soul's journey to a better place seemed so disingenuous. I just didn't want to be a witness to it. In any event, we primped and primed Mom for her last rendezvous with family and friends. She looked so serene in her white sari with brown edging, and I realized that I'd never seen her look so at peace. I suppose death does that to a person.

A couple of days after Mom left, my father called my phone. I didn't answer when I saw his number, so he left a message on my voice mail. I didn't listen to the whole message because I deleted it after I heard it's time to end this or something to that effect. I don't know what power he thought he had to end anything because I'd already ended it when I left him the letter. It was too late, and I had no interest in anything he had to say. The last time I saw my mother was in the funeral home, and a little over a year later, as I recounted my story to Philip, I still hadn't shed one tear for her leaving.

Philip was now up-to-date and asked how I felt about all of this. I told him I had forgiven my father because I didn't want to harbor any negative feelings about him since I believed it would give him power over me. I told him I'd read and I understood (even though I didn't have any proof) that souls make contracts with each other to learn specific lessons in the earthly realm, and if there was even a remote possibility this was how the world works, it was easy for me to forgive. I thought that if my mother and father had a contract with each other to learn life lessons, how could I possibly be angry with him? All he would have been doing was holding up his end of the deal. I may not have agreed with the way they lived their lives, because by the same token, there are infinite choices they could have made and things could have been very different.

Even though they were ultimately their lives to live, my parents' choices affected me in many ways. My belief that we are all on a spiritual journey and one of the ways we learn lessons is through interactions with the people in our lives, our family members being the most fundamental teachers, made it easy for me to forgive. I believed my parents were in a symbiotic relationship, fulfilling their spiritual promises to each other; this was my way of understanding their relationship with one another. Maybe they both didn't make the best choices, but who was I to judge? I said to Philip it was my way of dealing with the pain and trauma of seeing the violence I did as a child, and that it was the only way I knew how not to let my experiences devastate my life by holding on to anger and resentment.

Philip said that I'd dealt with the situation remarkably well, but he wanted to explore my childhood because I explained there was a part of me that wished I hadn't seen certain things while I was growing up. I said that I didn't necessarily blame anyone, and I accepted that it was what it was. I told him there was physical violence against Mom, along with emotional abuse, which, to me, was sometimes worse. Beating one's wife at that time was an unspoken, culturally accepted norm and I never really knew what any of the arguments were about, but understood that something was about to go down when I heard raised voices and a tone that indicated nothing good was coming. Like in any typical marriage, my parents argued. Then there were periods of tension in the home, and, quite naturally, things eventually went back to 'normal' until the next episode.

I told Philip that I'd spent a lifetime trying to deal with memories from my childhood every time my parents had marital issues because Mom confided in me. As much as I tried to have a happy life when I was finally able to live on my own, it was almost impossible to stay neutral because I still sort of experienced it along with her, even though I didn't live at home any longer.

The day I saw Mom with her black eye opened up a Pandora's Box of memories I'd tried to bury in a place so far in the recesses of my mind, I thought I would never think of them again. Seeing the sadness in her eyes that day triggered horrible memories; memories I'd tried to suffocate my whole life and was one of the reasons I couldn't continue to visit her at the house anymore. I couldn't help her, but I also couldn't be a witness to how my father treated her. One of the things that bothered me was how he made her perform. For instance, he would start a sentence of a nursery rhyme, like "Hickory Dickory," and wait for her to finish with "Duck," and he wouldn't stop until she responded. When she completed the sentence after his relentless badgering, he would laugh because he thought it was funny.

A friend of the family told me, two years after Mom left, that she felt he treated Mom like a show dog performing tricks and tried to persuade him many times that he shouldn't do it because it was embarrassing to Mom, even if she didn't know it. She said she felt sorry for Mom, but no amount of reasoning with my father made him stop. Trying to make him see how his actions were hurtful, even though he thought they were funny, was like trying to nail water to a wall. I don't understand and never will follow my father's thought processes, but it hurt to see how he treated her. One of his favorite things to do was make ugly faces and make loud snorting noises as she screamed and screamed until he got what he wanted, which was for her to laugh, which she ultimately did. Sometimes in these moments, I wondered if he did these things in someone else's presence, what did he do when no one was around?

I learned that the neighbors once called the police because they heard Mom's screams from inside the house and became concerned. Of course, it was explained that she had dementia, and she sometimes screamed. From what I witnessed, she screamed at the top of her lungs only on those occasions where she was displeased about something because it was the only way she knew how to communicate.

When Mom became nonverbal, she filled her days watching TV, or more often than not, in her bed, which I think was sort of a sanctuary for her. The most peaceful times we shared were when it was just the two of us together in her bed, and every time I drove to the house to see her, I prayed for these moments. As much as we all preferred that Mom not spend so much time in bed, she seemed to be much more at peace when she was there by herself. She didn't sleep, but I felt she had a sense of calm because no TV or computer was blaring at the same time.

However, if she was watching TV and my father was at home, I knew it would be uncomfortable. Most of the time, when I visited, his laptop was on a few feet away from Mom, blasting the online radio program.

It was something he had done many times when she was well, and she would plead with him to turn the volume down. When he ignored her, she would roll her eyes and let out a huge sigh.

I would joke with her, saying, "You hitched your wagon to that horse," trying to make light of the situation. She'd smile and say, "True," but I knew she felt discounted. This habit never changed, and there were many times I visited, and the computer volume was so disturbingly loud while she watched TV. The noise was annoying to me, and I couldn't even imagine what she felt like in her state of dementia. Many years ago, I volunteered at a call-in hotline for people with emotional issues who needed to speak to another human being. As part of the training, we did an exercise where I had four people (one to the back, one to the front, and one on either side of me), all talking to me at the same time.

The exercise helped the volunteers feel what callers who had schizophrenia felt like, so we understood how to deal with someone if they told us they had the condition. I felt this way when the TV and his computer were on at the same time. When I didn't think it could get worse, he would get on the phone and have a conversation, trying to talk above his computer and the TV.

There were times I visited, and Mom was home alone watching TV while his computer was on. There just didn't seem to be any compassion and understanding, or maybe his way of showing compassion was different. It amazed me how my father would spend time scouring websites looking for a deal. I wondered if he spent any time at all researching dementia or even diabetes, so he could better understand what Mom's specific needs were.

I told Philip this was all in my past, and I'd dealt with it. Since I was no longer a witness to it and hadn't been since I decided not to visit Mom anymore, I didn't think it affected me. He said that it was necessary to talk about my childhood experience to explore this anger and tension, which I possibly held in my body. I didn't think I was holding anything in my body because I thought I did a pretty good job of dealing with not only my childhood but also the last nine years of Mom's life.

But, Philip said talking about my past was key to my healing. I explained that I had lived all of my childhood and most of my adolescence and adulthood in fear of my father. It was a fear that permeated my mind and body even when things seemed to be okay because I always seemed to be waiting for the other shoe to drop. He ruled with a sort of intimidation that prompted fear in me at just hearing his footsteps at times. I must say that he wasn't always angry, and we did have happy times. My most wonderful memories were when we spent time at the beach with my cousins. However, I understood from a very young age that he viewed our behavior as children and Mom's as well as a personal reflection on him. He would admonish us not to "bring him shame" because we lived in a small community where he was well-known.

My earliest memory seeing my mother in physical pain occurred when I was about five or six years old, but I learned there was physical violence in the home when I was a young toddler. I am grateful my memories don't go that far back because it would add to the awful ones I have already. I was not present for what led up to this particular argument, which wasn't unusual, so I didn't know what was happening until I saw Mom running behind my father as he got into his car. She pleaded with him not to leave, and I remember his face, his nostrils flaring, and his breath quick as he angrily stomped to the car. As he started the engine, my mother held onto the car through the open windows and didn't let go as he drove off. I watched as she was dragged along the gravel road before she let go and slumped to the ground.

He drove off without even looking back and left her in a cloud of dust left behind by the whirling tires. I looked at her lying on the road, crying and bruised. I ran to her as she got up and made her way up the driveway, and when I looked into her eyes, I saw a kind of sadness, one I would see over and over again through the years. The look in her eyes and the sound of her voice, in emotional or physical pain, distressed me for most of my life. From that moment on, if I was not in the same room with my parents, and I heard her voice, and there was even a slight indication she was in pain (though it may have been only in my mind), my body trembled with fear.

I didn't want to get involved in my parents' marriage, but I don't know how much choice I had. The abuse was in plain sight, without regard or worry for the young eyes that observed it. Three children (seven, six, and four) slept crossways on one bed, even though there was another bedroom, and the baby slept in a crib in my parents' room. We went to bed one night, unaware of what the next few minutes would bring, as there was nothing in the air to demonstrate any sort of impending argument. My father was in the bathroom, and Mom was ironing his clothes. Out of the blue, there was shouting. I don't remember what was said, but the tone indicated trouble was brewing. As we lay in bed, listening to the shouting of my father from the bathroom, my body convulsed and trembled with fear because I knew something dreadful was about to happen.

Then the footsteps, so heavy I thought he would fall through the wooden floor of our old house. Their room connected to ours by a door, and I saw him sprint across the doorway in her direction, stark naked. We remained in bed, no one saying a word, and listened as the footsteps headed toward Mom. She began to shout and cry, and through her crying, I heard her say, "Get some clothes on! The children!" I was shaking uncontrollably by this time, and I saw him hurriedly walk back in the direction of the bathroom. All three of us jumped out of bed and rushed over to Mom. She was crying, holding the iron as she bled from a cut on her nose. The fear made me tremble and tense up, and it felt like my body was going to freeze where I stood.

When he headed back to the bathroom, I thought it was all over. All four kids, myself included, were hysterical and crying as we watched Mom bleeding. I don't know if the baby saw when Mom was hurt, but she was frantic and screaming. I ran to her, but of course, I couldn't get her out of her crib because the bars were just as tall as I was. As I tried to calm her, I heard the footsteps again, this time they were headed back toward us. I didn't know what would happen, and with my back turned as I tried to hush my baby sister, I heard a sound I couldn't decipher.

When I looked over my right shoulder, I saw my father straddling Mom on the bed, and it was then that I realized what the sound was—the sound of his fist as it connected with her face and a sound that came out of her! She didn't scream or yell; it was just a sound that she made each time he hit her. I didn't see how he'd managed, but he'd gotten her on the bed crossways, straddled her, and used his left hand to hold both her hands and pinned her down. I froze where I stood, and it felt like everything in me locked down when I tried to move. I felt like I was in a bad dream, where you are trying to run but can't. I watched as he repeatedly hit Mom's face with his fist, the sound causing a wrenching in my stomach, and I thought I would vomit. Even as he was hitting her, I heard her cautioning my father about the state of children.

I somehow managed to make my legs work and ran to Mom, whose face by this time was bloody. All three children were now screaming at the top of our lungs, begging our father to leave Mom alone, while the baby bawled in her crib. I stood so close to her, my entire body convulsing on the inside, and watched as he hit her repeatedly. When it didn't seem as though he would stop, I waited until his arm was up in the air, and I lay upside down on her at her head. I covered her face with mine and locked my little fingers around her neck. I could smell the combination of blood, tears, and her breath. I waited for his fist at the back of my head, but it didn't come. He may as well have hit me because every time I saw his fist connect with her face, I felt the pain in mine as well.

While I covered her face with mine, she said to me in a low voice, the kind your mother uses when she means business, "Move!"

I immediately responded, "No!" There was no way I was moving because I was sure that, as soon as I was off of her, he would hit her again. She again told me to move, ever so slightly louder and more forcefully this time. I was so torn because when she told you to do something, you automatically did it, no questions asked. I thought I would be able to protect her as long as I held my position over her face, but now I felt so powerless because I had to move! I was so close to her, looking into her eyes, and I saw her pain and fear. Just as I lifted my head away from hers, I saw his fist connect with her face again. While he was hitting her, she kept saying to him to look at the state of the children. It's hard to say how long this went on for, but in my seven-year-old mind, it felt like forever.

When he wouldn't stop with us three children hysterically begging him to leave Mom alone, I ran to the spare bedroom, where I had taped up a newspaper clipping of a Hindu goddess we'd seen in a religious movie, *Jai Santoshi Maa*. There was not much choice of entertainment in those days, so going to see this movie had been quite a treat. The characters in the film were in some dire distress and begged the goddess for help. She appeared before them in all of her magnificent glory and helped them out of their painful experience. Watching this on a big movie screen, with the accompanying dramatic musical score only added to the awe I felt. Jai Santoshi exuded such power and control, two things neither Mom nor I had at this moment.

To an impressionable seven-year-old brain, the intervention of this goddess seemed the only way my mother was going to get out from under my father. For sure, this was bad enough to warrant her assistance! I stood in front of the newspaper clipping with my hands clasped and prayed to the Goddess Santoshi to come down like she did in the movie and help Mom. I thought that if I could pray the way the characters did in the film, then the goddess would appear and stop this madness from happening. I'd never asked for anything in my short life with as much yearning and aching the way I asked for help that night. After what seemed like a lifetime of begging, pleading, and praying, I realized Santoshi was not going to appear like she did in the movie. *How could she not help us?* Then the anger! Anger at the goddess for what I felt was absolute abandonment.

I ran back to their bedroom, and he had finally had his fill and got up off of her, leaving her limp and weak. There aren't words to describe the depth of sadness I felt for Mom when I looked in her eyes, and the fear I felt as I watched my father, his nostrils flaring and his breath rapid with anger. After calming the baby, she rounded us up and took us back to our bed. I lay there, my body convulsing with fear, digesting what I had seen, heard, smelled, and felt. I couldn't stop shaking and trembling no matter how I tried, and the fear felt as if it were oozing through my pores. My neck locked up, and my insides quivered, and the more I tried to steady myself, the worse it felt. It was a sleepless night, as I waited in anticipation of another incident, but nothing happened.

I don't remember if it was the following morning or if it was a separate incident, but one morning there was another argument. I heard the tone in my father's voice and his heavy footsteps, and I trembled with fear but made myself move just in time to see him going for Mom. This time I decided I wasn't going to allow him to hit her again, so I ran to the kitchen and got the broom, determined to deter him. As fast as I ran back to them, ready to unleash my wrath on him, she yelled at me, "Aye, put the broom back in the kitchen!" stopping me dead in my tracks. Sheepishly, I listened, but I couldn't understand in my young mind how she could allow him to do what he was doing.

I realized that, for whatever reason, he wasn't going to hit me and wanted her to use that as leverage, but she just wouldn't. She fiercely protected her brood, even when her safety was in danger. The nightmare ended with him putting her out the back door in the kitchen while she was still in her nightgown. I stood defiantly watching him, as he put a plastic bag into the hole where the other side of the door's hook went in, to keep her from rattling the old estate-style door open. At that moment, I don't know if he saw in my eyes that I would do whatever I could to help her. I waited until he left the kitchen and opened the door to see Mom changing into clothes that hung on the clothesline. She made me go back into the house to get the younger ones ready, as we were leaving because he'd told her to get out and take her children with her.

We all got dressed, and I got the baby ready and met Mom at the front of the house. A long driveway led up to the house, and we all walked in silence down to the main road, not knowing where we were going. At the end of the driveway, she handed the baby to me and told us to wait that she was going to get a taxi. It seemed like hours we stood there, waiting on the side of the road until I looked up to the house and saw my father heading toward us. I started shaking uncontrollably again on the inside, fear gripping every organ, limb, and muscle of my body. I didn't know what I would do, as Mom told us not to move until she got back. I didn't know what his intention was, and I watched as he approached. She wasn't there to tell me not to stand up to him, so I was ready for anything. I decided I would certainly not allow him to do to me what I saw him do to her, remembering that horrible night, the memory causing a wrenching in my stomach.

I didn't think about our size difference and the inevitability of me losing a one-on-one fight with him. When he finally got to us, he casually handed each of us an apple and said, "Here, this is for your Christmas," and walked back to the house.

I am not sure if this happened on Christmas Day, but it was only around this time of the year that we got these apples as they were a seasonal delicacy. I stood there in absolute disbelief, holding my apple, my fear now turning to something else: anger! I was so angry at him! (It was at this moment in my and Philip's conversation that I realized I'd found the origin of the anger Tom had cautioned me about). As much as I tried, I couldn't understand how a father could see his four children, one just a baby, at the side of the road (possibly on Christmas Day), and the best he could do was give us each an apple and walk away. To this day, I can't eat that particular apple, and even the smell of it evokes the terrible memory of that day.

Mom returned with a taxi driver, and we went to one of her sister's home, where we spent the day. That night my cousins, siblings, and I were corralled into my uncle's van. The hour or so it took to get back to our house was nerve-racking, and I felt the same fear vibrating in my body. While the adults went to speak with my father, we waited quietly in the van. The fear that took over my body again made me sick, but I had no choice, as this was our home. I don't know what the discussion was, but we were let back into the house.

A few days later, my father's parents came to visit as they had heard what had happened. When we were growing up, we always heard adults say that children should be seen and not heard, and when adults were talking, children had to leave the room. Being inquisitive and curious, I wanted to listen to what the adults were saying. As quietly as I could, I began to eavesdrop—starting at the point in the conversation where I heard my grandmother say, "You all have children now, it is time to behave."

I was astounded! They had to behave?! What I witnessed was not mis-behavior! My mother had a cut on her nose, and he pounded her face with his fist! That was not misbehaving in my eyes. Children misbehaved, not parents!

Philip saw the physical effect our discussion had on me, as I shook my legs a mile a minute and wrung my hands. I don't know if he noticed, but I was shaking uncontrollably. He said we needed to take a break and should try an exercise to help the little girl who had witnessed this horrible act. He told me to close my eyes and go back to that night. I looked at him, my eyes almost falling out of my head because I couldn't understand why he wanted me to experience that horrible night again. I was having a difficult enough time just talking about it, and my stomach tensed up so much that it hurt more. But, he asked me to trust him.

I closed my eyes, and as he talked me through the exercise, I felt pure panic and fear take over my body! He told me to imagine that I had a time machine, and, to go back and visit the little girl who protected Mom that night. I had to leave her and go to the bedroom where the little girl prayed to the picture taped to the wall. I had to sit with her on the bed and hug her, comfort her, wipe her tears away, and reassure her that everything would be okay.

As I heard him say this, I thought to myself that this man must have taken leave of his proper senses, because no, it didn't turn out okay. My father beat the crap out of Mom. I fought the urge to express my thoughts and continued with the exercise, but he must have sensed my hesitation and reminded me in his soothing, reassuring voice to trust him. I did as he asked, and for a few minutes, I imagined holding the scared little girl in my arms, and I could feel her, and it felt so real. I felt her trembling tiny body and her fear as I held her and told her that it would all be okay.

I held her for what seemed to be a long time until Philip asked me if she felt better. I told him that yes, she did, and he told me to say to her that anytime she needed me, she just had to call on me, and I would be there for her. I did feel better after the exercise, and, for many nights after doing this with Philip, before I went to sleep, I visited that little girl in my time machine and held her until she told me she was okay.

At my next session with Philip, we talked about life after this incident. I said I didn't witness any more violent attacks like this against Mom, but my younger sister and brother were not spared. I am not sure why but my father never hit me. Maybe it was the defiance he saw in my eyes when situations were tense in the house.

I watched as he beat my younger sister for losing her textbook in primary school. When he picked us up from school, her teacher gave my father the news, and the ride home was pure hell. I knew, and I am sure she knew what was coming. As soon as he got out of the car, he pulled his belt off his waist. As she got onto the porch, he grabbed her by her wrist and started beating her. She ran in circles around him, screaming and crying as he continuously hit her with his leather belt, reprimanding her with every stroke about losing her book and how much money it cost. When I looked down at the green concrete floor of the porch, I saw spots and realized she had peed herself as she ran around him, making a circle with her drops of urine.

I trembled as I watched her in pain, but I couldn't help her, because how do you catch a moving target? I couldn't intervene because I was sure the belt would have connected with me had I tried to grab it, so we just stood there and watched as she screamed and cried, totally helpless and in pain.

I told Philip that my father beat my younger brother with a belt so severely one time that he was about to pass out before he finally listened to my mother, pleading with him to "look at the condition the child is in" and to let him go. My brother slumped to the ground, and Mom picked him up and took him to the bed and rubbed petroleum jelly on the welts on his body. I watched as my brother gasped as he tried to catch his breath from crying in utter physical pain, and I could only imagine the emotional terror he felt. I remember why my brother got the belt. Still, maybe a good talking to and an explanation about why his behavior was wrong, might have been more effective in preventing a recurrence of his conduct in the future. The beating didn't.

Even though I didn't get the belt, the possibility existed that I could be next, and as far as I was concerned, it was worse than the actual beating. My siblings probably wouldn't agree with me, but it's all about perspective. Don't get me wrong, I am grateful my father didn't beat me the way he did the others, but I lived with a constant fear that I could be next.

His anger knew no limits, and even though my sister and brother were the transgressors, anyone of us could have been his target for any misdemeanor. My body vibrated and shook with fear, watching the pain he inflicted on my family, and the possibility of him coming at me made me sick inside. The threat and fear of being beaten with a belt was excruciating and ever-present. For example, my father took our performance in school as a personal reflection on him and told our teachers to beat us if we needed it. I got the whip many times from my teachers in primary school, with his permission, because I was horrible in math.

At home, he would fold his belt in two, hold it by the buckle and end, and make me recite the multiplication tables. When I got stuck, he'd hit the belt over his shoulder and across his shirtless back, prompting me to flinch and sometimes pee a little. I remembered some, but mostly I didn't remember, and to this day, I am still horrible at math and freeze up if I have to do calculations in my head under pressure. The ironic thing was that I knew the answers, but remembering them with the threat of a belt or whip made me forget very quickly.

I knew how important it was to do well in school because bringing home a poor report card meant bringing shame to my father. I tried my best to be first in my class, but the position always eluded me, not because I wasn't smart, but because there was someone more intelligent. Students were graded based on the average grade of all subjects, and I could snag only third or fourth place. The trembling and shaking started when I got my report card in school and saw that I didn't come in first place. When he asked us to bring our report cards to him, fear gripped me, and I thought I would get the belt for sure because I didn't get the highest grade. He would read it, hold it between his middle and index fingers, and toss it at me, asking why I didn't come first in my class. I knew how important it was to my father that I did well in school, but my efforts felt as if they were all in vain, and nothing I did was good enough.

I spent my childhood, most of my adolescence, and even some of my adult life always seeking my father's approval and fearing that my actions would bring him shame. The act of writing this book would most likely be interpreted as me bringing him shame, as opposed to me expressing my absolute fear of him when I was growing up. I know him well, and he would never see it that way. After the bouts of violence against Mom, he blamed his actions on her, saying that she made him angry. No one spoke about the events after they happened, I assume, because we didn't want to rehash such horrible experiences.

Life went on, and I never thought about my experiences from my childhood until there was trouble in my parents' marriage, and Mom confided in me. I think it was in my fourth year at university when I had a reminder. I was on a subway train headed home after a long day. I had a long ride ahead of me and was already tired, so I rested my head against the window of the train and dozed off. Out of nowhere, a violent vision jolted me right out of my sleep, and I woke up frantic, not remembering where I was. I managed to collect my thoughts and remembered that I was on the subway. Then my mind went back to the vision of my father hitting my mother. It made me sick inside, and I knew something was wrong. My journey took almost two hours before I got home to the apartment I shared with my brother.

When I grabbed the door handle to open it, I felt it move before I could push it down. My brother pulled the door open in his direction, and before he could say anything, I said,

"He hit her, right?" He looked at me, surprised. "How did you know?" All I could say was that I just did. We immediately left for the hour drive north to my parents' home. The police had arrested my father because Mom had called the police. She was distraught, and even though she didn't give any details, I saw that same expression of utter humiliation, shame, and sadness in her eyes.

The next day she went to the courthouse, and I accompanied her. I saw my father sitting in the distance, and as I started toward him, I heard Mom say, defiantly, "Come here." I ignored her because I was going to have my say. I made sure to obey her never disrespect your father warnings, so I didn't use profanity when I spoke to him. I very coolly walked up to him, stood in front of him, and waited for him to acknowledge my presence. He looked at me up and down with pure contempt in his eyes, but I didn't give a rat's ass. I said to him in a low voice, "You feel like a big man now?" I wanted a response and waited with my eyes fixed on him.

The person who sat beside him, whom I presumed was his lawyer, asked who I was, and words I never thought I would hear fell from his lips: "My stepdaughter."

Even though my father didn't legally adopt my brother and me, I'd never heard those words uttered before, as he considered my brother and me his children. Friends of the family were considered uncles and aunts and respected accordingly. Cousins, though not related by blood, were deemed to be full cousins and treated no differently. Yet here we were.

He was in a court for domestic abuse, and I suddenly became the wicked stepchild. I was used to his deflection of responsibility, so I smirked and walked away without a word.

Mom later dropped the charges against him because she said she couldn't do it to him, meaning he would have a criminal record, and it would have negatively impacted his business. He tried to convince my sister, years later, that he had never hit Mom, but I don't believe him. I was not there, but I know something happened because it was too much of a coincidence that I'd had the intense vision I did when I was asleep on a train on the exact day of the incident.

Philip listened while I talked about this, and I could see the compassion in his eyes. He saw the physical effect our discussion had on me yet again, as I trembled and wrung my hands. My failed attempt to hide my chattering teeth showed my distress, and I knew he was observing me. I knew what he was thinking, but I couldn't stop myself from shaking. *Is anger making my body hurt this way?* It didn't make sense to me, but by the physical reaction I was having to our discussion, I realized that my childhood experiences were still affecting me, and I wanted to pursue it further.

Philip wanted me to do an exercise called EFT (Emotional Freedom Technique), which I'd had minimal exposure to a couple of years back but hadn't put much faith in, because the idea of 'tapping' to release emotions seemed strange to me. He said to follow his lead and repeat the words he said.

I went through the exercise and did feel some relief, not from the pain but the constant tensing and trembling in my body, which in effect made my pain worse. At our sessions, we did the EFT exercise when he recognized the signs of stress from talking about my childhood, and I learned to do the exercises at home with a bit of personal tweaking. I was so exhausted when I finished my sessions; all I could do when I got home was to collapse on the sofa for a couple of hours.

We continued our conversations about Mom and what I'd observed. As we got older, and maybe as he got older too, my father probably realized he couldn't physically beat anymore. The physical abuse tapered off, but the emotional terrorism remained. The constant warnings that we better not bring him shame ensured that we lived according to his rule. We already knew what he was capable of, so we lived in constant fear of him. It wasn't always horrible, as there were times we did have fun and laughed. I would not say my entire life was terrible, but the undertones always seemed to permeate even when things were good.

When I was a child, Mom didn't talk to me about her pain, I presume because I was so young, but she didn't have to, because I could see it in her eyes. As I matured, however, she relied on me more and confided her feelings and fears, and sometimes it was a heavy burden to bear. In my twenties, the responsibility got to be too much, and I started to show signs of stress when she shared her feelings about their marital problems with me. The physical symptoms, like hives, were terrible, but the emotional turmoil was worse, as I experienced depressive states and found it hard to cope since I was away and couldn't help her. I also had my survival to worry about because I had to support myself while I attended university.

I had to figure out a way to deal with my parents' problems because they had started to affect my life. I didn't know where else to turn, so I sought the help of a psychiatrist. I had just one session with the female doctor, who I became enraged at when she told me, "It's your mother's life, not yours." I never went back to her because I felt like she didn't know what Mom endured, and therefore had no right to say what she did. After thinking about it for a few days, I agreed with her statement, but I still couldn't figure out how not to be involved. I felt like I was all she had.

It was after her passing that I understood and cherished her confidence in me. After talking to one of her best friends, who was like a sister to her, as well as to her sister (both of whom I thought were close confidants), I realized they knew nothing about her deep pain.

Mom was devoted to her marriage and her children, and she did the best she could. I believed, for most of my life, that even my father did the best he could. It was a coping tactic that I think I adopted because I didn't want to believe that he could do better yet deliberately chose to act the way he did with his family. I struggled with this, however, when I heard him multiple times on the phone, giving people advice about their domestic issues. I was always amazed at how he seemed to understand how people should be treated, yet did the complete opposite in his own home.

He was charming and loving to people on the outside, but when it came to showing affection within the home, he seemed incapable. My mother was deeply hurt about this and felt responsible because she thought she couldn't do anything to change how he treated us. I chalked up my father's inability to show love in his home, to his childhood and convinced myself that I was being understanding and empathetic.

I explained to Philip that, regardless of my childhood, I decided to focus on the times I did feel happy, as well as the times I saw my parents happy.

Philip suggested we try an exercise to deal with what was evident to him but not to me: my repressed psychological pain. He had a broken foot and was in his wheelchair when I came in for my sessions, so he asked me to place a chair in front of me and pretend that my father was sitting in it. I had to have a conversation with him, as if he sat in front of me, about what I'd felt in those moments when I witnessed violence, not only against Mom but my siblings as well.

In my mind, I didn't think my childhood experiences and the years leading up to Mom's passing contributed in any way to my physical pain, because Philip had said I'd handled things remarkably well. I thought I had done everything right by being forgiving and understanding, so why did I have to go through this seemingly worthless exercise? I thought it made no sense because it was never going to happen in real life, and besides, I'd moved on. However, in the spirit of exploring my psychological pain and its possible ties to my physical pain, I went along with him.

I spoke from where I sat to my pretend father, who sat in the chair in front of me, looking into what I believed would be his eyes, never letting go of his gaze. I wasn't prepared for what I felt as I spoke to my father about how I felt when I saw him pounding my mother's face with his fist. I didn't think it was possible to feel precisely the same emotions I had more than forty years ago, but I did. I wrung my hands, and my stomach and chest felt like something was squeezing the very life from me. I went from being cold (which I always seemed to be) to being hot and had to take off my jacket because I started to sweat. My body shook just like it did when I was a child, and my neck, stomach, and sides tightened up. I felt like I'd had lost all control.

I told my father that he was responsible for me being the way I was right now, in pain, hysterically crying, and totally out of control. I told him that he was supposed to protect me, not be the reason I was scared out of my mind. I told him that he made me feel small, worthless, and insignificant as if nothing I did ever pleased him. I told him that I was scared for myself and everyone in the house and that this fear had followed me my whole life.

When I couldn't talk anymore through the frantic crying, Philip waited a few moments and asked me to switch places. Now I had to pretend to be my father, responding to everything I'd just said. It was incredible to me how I unconsciously sat the way he sat, and as I realized this, it dawned on me that it didn't matter that my father wasn't sitting in front of me, listening to how much pain he'd caused me for most of my life.

As him, I responded to the empty chair in front of me, which was me, and said, "I don't see why you have to bring this up. That's all in the past, and it's time to get on with your life!"

I couldn't believe the words coming out of my mouth but caught myself and again realized that this is what he would say if we did have this conversation. He was never one to take responsibility for his actions. I then switched seats and became me again, to respond to what he said, and I tried again to make him understand the effect his actions had had on me. It was interesting that, when I was me, I shook and tensed up as I spoke to him, but when I imagined myself as him, I didn't. My body felt different, and it was then that I understood the power of this exercise and appreciated it more when I switched and became him again.

In response the second time (as him), I bowed my head in shame and said, "I'm sorry. I didn't know any better!" After a few moments passed, as him I said, "I have no excuse for my behavior, and I'm sorry for all I've done to hurt you, but I just didn't know better." As the words fell from my lips, I felt myself becoming angry because I felt as if I'd let him off the hook. There was now an inner war of emotions. Part of me felt compassion for him, and part of me felt angry at myself for what seemed like another excuse I was making for him. Even though compassion was the last thing I wanted to feel for him at that moment, I somewhat believed what I was saying; I honestly thought he was sorry for his actions, and he didn't know better.

When I became me again, somehow, something shifted in me. The shivering stopped, and I felt my body relax. The tears stopped flowing, and I sat like a bump on a log, spent, and exhausted. There were more emotions than we had time to deal with, and we had only a few minutes left in the session and did some EFT to release the stress from the exercise.

After every session with Philip, little by little, I felt a weight lifting off of me, but my physical pain persisted. I told him I couldn't believe I had this physical reaction to something that had happened such a long time ago. And even worse, I thought I'd dealt with it by being forgiving, blah blah blah.

He tilted his head to one side, looked me square in the eyes, and in a soft, low voice, he slowly responded, **"The mind may forget, but the body doesn't forget."**

I let what he said sink in for a few moments and then had an *AHA* moment because I'd convinced myself that I'd dealt with my childhood the way I was supposed to. Philip explained that all the negative emotions of fear and anger from my past experiences were bottled up inside and never got a chance to be resolved. I remembered my quantum healing hypnosis (QHHT) with Andrea, and contemplated her cautioning that I might have PTSD. When she said that no child comes out unscathed who'd witnessed what I had, I didn't take her all that seriously, because PTSD is something I thought only former soldiers experience. Also, I thought I'd done a pretty good job of dealing with my past. Yet here I was!

Every time there was an incident, my mother drilled it into my head that I should never hate my father. And I don't think I ever did. Most of my life, I made many excuses for his behavior. For instance, I said that maybe he had too much responsibility at a young age because he took my brother and me as his own. When I was a young teen, I was mesmerized on Saturday evenings when we watched *Little House on the Prairie* while my mother baked bread. I was captivated by the relationship

Charles and little Laura Ingalls shared, and I always envisioned that one day, my father and I would have the kind of father-daughter relationship, perhaps not like Charles and Laura, but one where I could feel safe and not always so afraid.

I was forty-one years old before I came to terms with the fact that it would never happen and gave up on the idea, yet I still appreciated him for all he did for me. The closest relationship my father and I had was when I moved to Trinidad to open a computer school with my brother. My brother worked in another country and funded the business and was supposed to join me after a year. The first time I heard my father say I love you on the phone, I almost dropped it. I didn't know how to respond, because, in my nearly thirty-something years on earth, I'd never heard the words before. They sounded very strange to me. Even though I'd had the experiences I did as a child, I never doubted his love for Mom or any of his children. I equated always having food, clothes, books for school, and a roof over our heads as his way of demonstrating his love.

If I met my father as a stranger, I probably would like him because he is charming and likes to have fun. He would do anything to help someone in need and give what he could. If he showed me the person I knew at home, however, I would quickly see we were very different people, and because I didn't share his views on almost everything, we probably wouldn't have a relationship. As I matured and understood him as a person, I'm sad to say I contemplated not having him in my life, but that was impossible because it meant giving up Mom.

He is the only father I know as I didn't grow up with my biological father, and I respected and loved him as such. As much as he is entitled to his beliefs and opinions, they have been in total opposition to mine. For instance, one time I was visiting Mom in her state of dementia, and as she and I sat in the living room, he was at the kitchen table listening to his radio program on his computer. The call-in program had caller after caller giving their racist views about Black children not doing as well as East Indian children in school because they were genetically inferior. The vitriol in their voices was revolting! He chuckled as the callers passionately spewed their hate, and with every call, I felt more and more disgusted. As if listening to this garbage wasn't enough, he got on the phone with a friend and repeated the callers' views, snickering and sneering, saying, "I'm not saying it, but you can see the truth."

I opened my mouth twice to say something to him but held back for two reasons: I knew it would have escalated into an argument, and nothing would get resolved, and I knew Mom understood everything happening around her. Even though she couldn't tell me to shut up this time because she couldn't talk, I didn't want her to see me going against her wishes and disrespecting my father.

Perspectives and beliefs like these made me not want to be around my father because I don't subscribe to his racist ideology. I believe everyone is entitled to their opinion on any given subject, but this one was personal, as ALL of his grandchildren so far have an African heritage. He didn't realize how hurtful his words could be and how close to home it was, and I concluded (as usual) that he was just clueless. Not to put words in his mouth, but he would probably justify his viewpoint by explaining that, since his grandchildren are 'mixed' (or some other ridiculous reasoning), these statements didn't include his loved ones.

I had to keep reminding myself that I couldn't counter intolerance with more intolerance, and I decided to go with compassion instead, for him and his foolish beliefs. I had no choice because he is one of those people you can't have a conversation with, hoping to get him to see how this type of thinking is hurtful to others. I know, for fact, that he wouldn't have a conversation of this nature with his son-in-law, daughter-in-law, or his grandchildren present, so why he thought it was okay to have it at all was beyond my understanding.

Sometimes life presents us with opportunities to learn, but despite that, even when it's right in front of our noses, we still are oblivious to the chance of redeeming ourselves. All things being equal, I probably would be able to ignore the way he processed things and say he was just quirky. For example, one day, I was making myself a salad and asked if he wanted one, because he was always on some diet, trying to lose weight. I told him that my salad had all kinds of goodies, like chickpeas and so on, and that it was good for him.

He said no, and even though we weren't discussing weight loss or dieting, he went on and on about people thinking that, because they eat salads, they will lose weight, and they were stupid for thinking this way. He backed up his theory that eating salads was nonsense, because, "how come cows are fat and all they eat is grass?" I paused for a few seconds, and my jaw dropped in utter disbelief because it was arguably the stupidest thing I'd ever heard. I didn't think getting into a discussion with him about cows' natural girth would make sense, so I didn't continue my conversation with him. There was nothing I could say to refute this senseless argument, and I knew my father enough to know that it would be a fruitless exercise. In my mind, I secretly thought that maybe he was joking and left it at that.

We are very different people with different ideologies, but I tried to appreciate the good parts of him, as I genuinely believe we are all innately good. After his last warning to me about my brother's dishonesty, when I finally took his advice and walked away from the business in Trinidad, I had nowhere to go but right back into the family home with him and Mom. One thing I have learned about fear is that the very thing you fear the most always finds you wherever you are, as if to say, I am here … deal with me!

When I left home at eighteen, my biggest fear was that someday I would end up back at home with my parents, and that's what happened. However, I will always be grateful that he took me in because I had $800 to my name (from selling my belongings) and nowhere else to go.

When I was in Trinidad, he sold a piece of property he owned there and gave the money to my brother and me to get a property of our own. He said that since we had a business, we would someday want our own homes, and the money would be a sort of starter fund. After I moved back to Canada, it took over three years to get the funds transferred from the investment fund in Trinidad wired to me. I tried to return it to my father because I felt that the intended purpose for which he gave the money did not materialize. He said that he had given it to us, and it was ours to keep, and it was all he had to offer, and I appreciated his goodwill. I got a draft for half the amount after it I converted into Canadian dollars and left it for my brother.

It seemed as though it was easier for my father to be expressive the further away I was. I don't know why, and don't want to make assumptions and be wrong, because only he knows (maybe) why it was easier to have a good relationship when I was far away. In any case, I appreciated him and all he did for me. When I moved back into their home just before my fortieth birthday, I realized, after not living at home since I was eighteen, not much had changed. I never again heard the words I'd been hearing on the phone for the five years I was away, but I viewed his helping me get back on my feet as love enough and appreciated him.

I stayed with my parents for a little under two years and saw the same old patterns of behavior. When the opportunity presented itself for a job away from home, I took it as fast as I could. I got a job, with Kathryn's help, at the company she worked with, and she and her roommate put me up in the small apartment they rented while they awaited the completion of their condo. When they left, I took over the lease, and this is where things took a turn for the worse. By May of that year, Mom left her home and came to live with me when she found out her husband had contacted an old girlfriend. My relationship with my father only got worse as time went by, and he has not been in my home since I've lived on my own (over ten years).

I live with questions that sometimes I think I don't want the answers to because they could disrupt the sense of peace I got with Mom's leaving. Trust is something I believe is earned, and once someone breaks that trust, it's hard to get it back. Once, Mom had an appointment with the Aging Well Clinic, and Kathryn was supposed to accompany her and my father. Close to the appointment time, my father called Kathryn to tell her the clinic had called and cancelled the appointment, saying the nurse practitioner had a family emergency.

I called the clinic because I had a gut feeling it wasn't true and spoke with the nurse practitioner. She said that he was the one who'd called and cancelled the appointment, and didn't give a reason. I told her he'd said they cancelled and why, and she told me it wasn't true. There was no family emergency, and the fact that I was talking to her meant she was at the clinic. I couldn't ask him why he cancelled Mom's appointment, but I had an uneasy feeling about the whole thing and couldn't understand why he'd said what he did. If he couldn't make the appointment, he didn't have to explain anything more than to say something came up, and he needed to reschedule. To say they cancelled the appointment and give a reason when they didn't was odd and a tad bit suspicious.

On another visit to see Mom, I heard she had a doctor's appointment, but my sister, who was to accompany Mom, acted a bit peculiar. I didn't ask anything until she finally said she was meeting our father at a lawyer's office, as he had asked her to be a witness to a Power of Attorney document Mom was going to sign.

I said, "But Mom can't read or write, and why does he need a POA? He is her legal guardian."

I understood that, as they were legally married, he had full authority to make all decisions regarding Mom's care and anything else. She said he needed two witnesses and that he'd also asked my youngest brother, who was oblivious as to any of the happenings. While she was still at the house, my brother texted her and asked where and what time they had to meet, and she didn't respond in time, hoping he wouldn't make the meeting because she felt too uneasy.

She asked me what I thought she should do, and I told her she should do what her gut told her to do.

I don't know why my father felt that he needed a POA when he was legally Mom's guardian. My sister left, noticeably upset, after talking to her husband, who told her not to get involved as it didn't make sense to him either. She met our father at the lawyer's office, and my spidey senses were on full alert that something wasn't right. The result was that he never got his POA because when he met her, the lawyer realized Mom was not legally capable of signing a legal document and refused to go through with the POA. I heard my father asked about using her fingerprint, but the lawyer did his job, and there was no POA. The question I will always have is why he felt he needed a POA. No one was challenging his decisions regarding Mom because we all knew he did what he wanted.

Even though I appreciate my father for raising me as his own and for his financial assistance, unlike my mother, I don't have a blind, misguided sense of obligation to him, which would make me endure his ill-treatment for the rest of my life. Some may believe I am ungrateful for choosing not to have a relationship with him, but to those people, I say don't judge me if you haven't walked my path. I don't want to use terms like toxic—okay, guess I just did—but it's a matter of respect for myself. There is no justification for the way he treated me, just because I helped Mom, and if I had to do it over again, I probably would make the same choices. Maybe he would have felt better if she went to a shelter again, but I just didn't know how to let her. I feel robbed of the last three years of her life because I lived in constant fear of being cut off from seeing her. Observing from a broader perspective, however, I came to terms with it and know in my heart that she is only a thought away, and all of the earthly physical stuff that transpired will eventually be moot, maybe even amusing.

At another session with Philip, I dealt with the betrayal of my brother in much the same way and was surprised again by my body language when I 'became' him. I told him how hurt I was that he'd lied to and manipulated me for such a long time. I told him that, if he had other plans, all he had to do was let me know instead of leading me on for so long with such dishonesty, even after I questioned him multiple times. I told him how stupid I felt for falling for his lies, and he must have thought at the time that I was the daftest person alive to believe him consistently for so long. I told him that, deep down, I knew he was lying, even though I didn't have proof. I told him how his lies destroyed relationships I had with people, because of what he told them about me, saying things like, "there were inconsistencies in the books," which essentially translates to I had stolen money from the business.

When I switched places and became him to respond to me, I was very aware of the change in my body language. This time I unconsciously folded my arms tightly across my chest, sat straight up with my chest puffed out as I pretended to be him, speaking to me. Philip noticed it too and explained the body language of folded arms as a protective mechanism someone may adopt to insulate themselves because they feel vulnerable. He reminded me that my brother experienced the abuse first hand, unlike me, who just observed it and if only seeing it affected me so strongly, imagine how it affected him. I hadn't considered this perspective before, and I entered a new place of understanding.

My last words to my brother before I walked away from the business, the money in the investment account, and my entire life savings I had invested, were, "We need to talk!"

I said this as he ran down the stairs of the computer center, and his response was, "I don't have time for this. I have a plane to catch."

My friend Haydn, who I've known for over thirty-four years, and without whose help, I wouldn't have been able to complete the project, warned me multiple times during those five years. He interacted with my brother, and said to me many times, that something didn't make sense; and he didn't think my brother was being honest with me. I met someone who helped when we relocated the training center, and after spending fifteen minutes chatting alone with my brother, he pulled me aside and warned me to be careful.

When I asked what I needed to be careful about, he responded, "Your brother doesn't consider you the way you consider him." I asked what gave him that feeling, and he said there wasn't anything specific, but it was just the way he spoke, and I had to "read between the lines."

My brother doesn't realize how much I know. The depth of his deception was so endless, and it continued long after I walked away from the business, and even after he closed it. The subject matter would fill a whole separate book! But, contrary to my feeling like an idiot after it was all said and done, my intuition (from the beginning) and our parents were right, but hindsight is always 20/20. Being right, however, doesn't matter, and even though it was a long and painful process, I have made peace with my experiences. I then made a conscious decision about living life differently by not continuing to do what my family does when one's actions hurt another, which is to act as if nothing is wrong while issues never get resolved.

Yes, I dealt with my hurt, anger, and resentment, but I decided not to pretend, even for the sake of being part of a family, because something had changed in me that won't allow me to live the way I learned when I was growing up. I decided to change what I call the ostrich syndrome and stop burying my head in the sand and carrying on as if everything is all right while avoiding family issues just because they are unpleasant.

Just as an aside, ostriches put their heads in the sand to turn their eggs, which assures the very survival of their young and not to avoid unpleasantness, but you get my meaning.

My emotional healing started when I took responsibility for my thoughts and reactions to the experiences I had with my brother, understanding that none of his lies changed the essence of who I truly am. (Mom was right, as long I as I know the truth.) Our interaction has taught me this lesson, and I appreciate it for what it is. With this recognition, I then felt that I didn't need an apology from either my father or brother, as I already 'got' one from both when I had my sessions with Philip.

In my mind, when I imagined speaking to them about how their actions hurt me when I assumed their personality and apologized on their behalf, their apology was more than enough for me. I realized that I didn't need either of them to be present for me to complete my circle of hurt, apology, and forgiveness, as I believe we all make mistakes. I use the word mistake loosely because I also contemplate the possibility that there are no mistakes in life. If I didn't have the interactions with my brother and father, I wouldn't have had the resulting experiences that gave me opportunities to learn more about myself and certain choices and decisions about life.

As I write this book, it's been twelve years since I've spoken to my brother, though I have learned never to say never, so I won't say we will never have a relationship. Distancing myself from my brother as well as my father, is a choice I make, not out of anger or because I don't love them, but because I couldn't allow their behavior to continue. For a long time, I used to want them to acknowledge that their actions hurt me, but I realized that I would be holding myself in a kind of energetic mess with them, with a need to be right. I decided to acknowledge my part in our interactions and appreciate our potential spiritual contracts with each other, and more importantly, take the space I need for my healing.

After many years of giving lip service to the phrase, it's not my business what someone else thinks about me, good or bad, I decided to live it. My job is to hold a mirror up to my true self and be happy with (or at least understand) the choices and decisions I made, which were not always good for me. I also had to let others off the hook because I realized that the only person I should hold to my high standards is me. It took me a long time, but I now believe that, if my brother truly feels the means justified the end and his conscience is clear and allows him to live with his actions, then so be it. I have to do it differently than Mom did because I have more of a choice than she felt she had. Dealing with it the way she did, I believe, results in negative emotional dis-ease, which ultimately has physical consequences.

My choice not to have a relationship with them will maybe allow them time to complete their circles, and the option is up to them to choose what they do.

I remember watching an *Oprah Masterclass* when Pastor T.D. Jakes was a guest. He asked if someone stood next to you and stepped on your toe, and you said, "You stepped on my toe," and the person didn't acknowledge it, but continued to step on your toe, what would you do. Would you keep standing there, so they could keep stepping on your toe? Or would you move out of their reach so that they couldn't step on your toe? I decided to stand up for myself and not allow the behavior to continue. I finally realized it was time to move out of their reach to save my toes.

I continuously remind myself of something I read in Robert Schwartz's book that says,

> *Your greatest challenges are never what other people do, but rather about how you respond. They are about whether you can accept, understand, and thus rise above the emotions that others' actions cause you.*[4]

As much as this helped me get over the emotions of anger, resentment, and feeling like a fool, I still sometimes wondered if I made the right choice about not having a relationship with my brother. I got my answer when I was visiting Mom at the house one day, and I heard a conversation he had with Mom's caregiver. It confirmed I'd made the right decision because he didn't seem to grasp the weight and consequences his words could have. What he said to her caregiver regarding Mom's medical history left me in total awe at his skewed and bizarre relationship with the truth. I was with Mom in her bed, and he was downstairs, and I heard him tell Mom's caregiver that Mom's mother, her aunt, and her sister all had dementia.

I said to Mom, "You hear the stupidness your son is saying?" Even though she couldn't talk, she just looked at me, raised her eyebrows, and smiled. It was the furthest thing from the truth, as my grandmother died of a ruptured ulcer not long after he was born. She lived a considerable distance from the hospital, and by the time she arrived, it was too late. I don't know who told him Mom's aunt had dementia, but I asked a couple of people from Mom's generation, and they all said the same thing: "Not that I know of."

Mom's sister had a brain aneurysm, which left her with an occasional stutter during conversations, as she tried to remember what she wanted to say. But even though it took some time, she mostly got it out. When I lived in Trinidad, I spent time with my aunt, and she had no signs of dementia. Mom happened to be on vacation visiting me when my aunt transitioned, and we were both at the hospital the day she passed from complications due to diabetes.

My brother's lies wouldn't have mattered much at this point because they no longer affected me, but he gave false information to Mom's caregiver, who most likely reported it to her supervisor because the caregivers took notes every day they provided care for Mom. I'm sure they would've deemed this information relevant to her diagnosis and care. I'm aware there are different perceptions of truth, as ten people can have the same experience, and there is a possibility that all may recall it differently. A perception of fact, however, is entirely different. The fact is my grandmother did not have dementia, and neither did her sister or her other daughter.

Dementia did not run in our family, as he stated to Mom's caregiver. I've had a lot of exposure to my brother's untruths, and it always amazes me how he lies for the silliest of things that had no consequence to anything one way or the other. I don't think truth should be subjective, and to say something that is an outright untruth or give a perspective that distorts the original fact is questionable at best. On many occasions, I was caught in the middle of it, trying to figure out in seconds what I should say when someone asked me about something he'd told them that I knew wasn't true.

I firmly believe that people shouldn't morph truth or facts for their convenience, and it has always bothered me that he lies for no apparent reason. I assume he believes the things he says; otherwise, he wouldn't say them, but it still doesn't make them real. Those who didn't know better would take the information he gave at face value, but for me, it was too much work always having to decipher if what he said was true or not.

In my journey to find peace after my experience with my brother, I remember a compelling story in Eckhart Tolle's book, *A New Earth: Awakening to Your Life's Purpose*, which helped me to understand the importance of letting go of negativity and eased my anger toward him.

> *Two monks, Tanzan and Ekido, were walking along a country road that had become extremely muddy after heavy rains. Near a village, they came upon a young woman who was trying to cross the road, but the mud was so deep it would have ruined the silk kimono she was wearing. Tanzan at once picked her up and carried her to the other side. The monks walked on in silence. Five hours later, as they were approaching the lodging temple, Ekido couldn't restrain himself any longer. "Why did you carry that girl across the road?" he asked, "We monks are not supposed to do things like that."*
>
> *"I put the girl down hours ago," said Tanzan. "Are you still carrying her?"*[5]

Tolle says to imagine what life would be like for someone who lived like Ekido all the time, unable or unwilling to let go internally of situations, accumulating more and more "stuff" inside. You get a sense of what life is like for the majority of people on our planet.

This story helped me put my brother and father down because I just didn't want to carry the load of the pain either of them caused me any longer.

As I said before, I do believe unresolved emotions can lead to the physical manifestations we call disease in the body. If this is what happened to me, even though my sessions with Philip helped me deal with the violence and trauma in my life, I was far beyond a psychotherapeutic healing. There was so much more I needed to talk to Philip about, but I ran out of time. I had excruciatingly painful physical symptoms, and if I didn't find out what was causing them, it would eventually be disastrous. This much I knew.

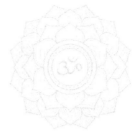

PHYSICAL JOURNEY

omething was awry in my body, and it required physical investigation. I stopped seeing Philip and turned my attention to looking for the monster that was slowly taking my life away. The pain in my left and right sides, as well as both arms, was so excruciating, I couldn't sleep on either side. I couldn't find a comfortable position on my back because when my head rested on the pillow, the pressure made it feel as though there was a line of fire from the base of my skull to my outer ear lobes.[1] The constant pulsating and pounding sensation persisted twenty-four hours a day, and I was able to withstand it during the day when my head and body weren't in contact with a surface. Sometimes simply walking up the stairs made the pounding so bad it sounded as if someone was knocking on my skull with their knuckles. When I was in bed, however, I felt the pulsating rhythm in my chest, neck, head, jaw, cheeks, and the erratic pounding in my stomach. Undeniably, the worst of it was when it felt like my entire brain, especially at the back of my head was vibrating with the tremors.[2] The sensation of my brain quivering made me feel as though I was losing my mind, and there are no words to explain what I felt like in those moments.

If I was able to ignore the pain and the horrible sensitivity to anything that touched my skin, the endless thumping in my ears when I tried to

---

1   See Notes for image showing the auricular branch of the vagus nerve.
2   See Notes for image showing the reach of the vagus nerve on the surface of the brain.

sleep on my side was so irritating that I just couldn't relax. For months, hours after going to bed, I would finally give up trying to sleep and stack some pillows behind my back and sit upright. This way, I could only feel the pounding in my chest and stomach, but couldn't hear the beat in my head or feel it in my neck and face. I spent anywhere from three to five hours, crying in pain and frustration because I just didn't know what else to do.

At my last physiotherapy session with Tom, he'd thought that I needed to check my stress levels, and suggested I go to a walk-in clinic, again, and demand a cortisol test. I don't consider myself a demanding person, but I was so desperate for answers that I thought I would give it a try. He thought that maybe my ongoing stress, which in part contributed to my TMJ, might also be a contributing factor to the pain in my sides because my adrenals were stressed.

The new information garnered from my sessions with Philip made me consider the possibility that, if Tom was right, maybe my pain was caused by the stress I'd endured for so many years, and especially the last three years before Mom's passing. I went to my local walk-in clinic for the third time and met Dr. Nancy, who seemed intrigued by the symptoms I described to her. I explained how long I'd had the pain and how it had spread and intensified. As she took my blood pressure, she enquired about any other symptoms that caused concern, and I mentioned that from January to May of that year, I lost approximately twenty-two pounds. Her eyes opened wide, and I could see her concern as she asked, "Without trying?" I said that I hovered between 135 and 145 pounds for most of my adult life, and I thought it was a healthy weight for me, so yes, it was without trying.

I remembered why I was there, and as she feverishly typed on her computer, I told her I wanted to have a cortisol test.

She retorted, "Aaaccchhhh, that's not a thing!" without even asking me why I thought I needed a cortisol test. She was concerned about the sudden and quick weight loss and said that she was signing me up for a cancer program at the hospital, where they would do "every test in the book."

My heart dropped to my feet as I heard the C-word. "Wait … what?!" I said, "Cancer? But how? What do you mean?" I was struggling for words. I wanted an answer to the pain I'd had for over a year, but cancer?! She said that anything was possible, and though she didn't think it was cancer, she felt that, whatever it was, they would find it at the cancer program, as it was a teaching program, and they were hungry (for knowledge.)

I felt a little relieved as I heard this, and she backed up her statement with statistics that said only 16 percent of people who went to the SOC clinic had cancer. Okay, my odds sounded pretty good, but still, cancer? Up until now, I had not even considered the weight loss an immediate threat to my health. I just saw myself in the mirror and knew I was losing weight, as my legs and arms got thin, with the accompanying sagging skin. As horrible as it looked and even though I was concerned, weight loss seemed a secondary issue that warranted less attention, and I hadn't put the two together at all.

In May of 2018, I went to the SOC (suspicion of cancer) Clinic for an initial consultation and met with the intern who listened attentively to my symptoms. He asked me to describe how my pain had started, took notes, and said that he needed to examine me. Getting on the examination table was difficult, as I couldn't bear much weight on either arm, the left one being worse. He did his examination, said he would be back shortly, and left to get the attending doctor.

William and I waited for the doctor, and, as he held my hand, I wondered if he was thinking the same thing I was thinking: *Cancer?!* He reassured me that everything would be okay, and we both felt relieved because Dr. Nancy had said, "Whatever it was, they will find it."

We were both comforted by the idea that they would keep searching until they found what the issue was, and I could finally get some help. Dr. Mukta came in after almost half an hour. She was a lovely lady, and we went over the same questions the intern had asked. She said that her assistant would set up the tests I needed, and it would happen relatively quickly, as cancer patients were a priority. At the end of the meeting, William asked Dr. Mukta if she could prescribe something for my pain since I got no relief with over-the-counter medications. She said that I had to go back to my family doctor because she couldn't prescribe anything. I didn't bother since I had already given up on him being of any help since he'd told me I had IBS.

We headed back to the car full of new hope. By this time, walking was quite challenging, as my left hip flexor locked up at the most inopportune times. My knees hurt, especially the left one. At times, as long as I was walking, I was okay, but when I stopped, my left leg would give out. The stitch in my sides and under my last set of ribs was so bad that holding myself up straight or sitting caused agonizing pain. Walking on my treadmill had now dwindled to 1.5 mph, and I was barely able to make twenty minutes because of the pain. I kept at it because I felt my legs beginning to feel like my arms, and I didn't want to lose my ability to walk. It felt as if there was not enough skin to cover the sole of my left foot, so it felt like it pulled whenever I walked.

Within two days, the SOC Clinic Patient Navigator called to set up appointments for a CT scan of the chest, abdomen, and pelvis, a bone scan; a skeletal survey; and blood work. Dr. Nancy also set up an appointment for an ultrasound of my heart because of the constant pounding.

I wore a heart monitor for forty-eight hours and recorded incidents as they happened, along with the time of day. Doing breathing exercises or meditation to control the pounding didn't work and seemed to make it worse. It woke me sometimes three to four times during the night when I was able to fall asleep finally. Sometimes, when I turned in my sleep (which caused pain), it made the pounding so much worse that I felt it in my jaw, teeth, and cheeks. Sometimes it felt as if I had many hearts all beating at different times, which resulted in confusing rhythms in my body. It was challenging to go back to sleep when this happened, and whatever sleep I managed to get was broken. I was so confused and didn't know who I could tell this to who wouldn't think I was crazy. (Little did I know!)

We waited anxiously for the results from the SOC Clinic, the heart monitor, and ultrasound. As the symptoms and pain got worse by the day, so did my anxiety, which made my heart pound even more. All I wanted was to find out what the issue was and deal with it. I was so frustrated with the medical doctors, but also at myself for getting sick, and I just wanted to get on the road to recovery and forget the last thirteen months.

The call finally came that my test results were in and to book the follow-up appointment. On our drive to see Dr. Mukta, I felt a combination of hope and fear. I was hopeful they had found something, anything, even cancer, to explain the sort of pain I was having, where sometimes it felt as if someone was hammering on my bones. I don't mean I wanted them to find cancer, but I was so desperate for an answer, I thought I could deal with anything as long as I knew what it was because I couldn't fight a ghost. I knew William would be by my side, so I was ready for anything.

On the other end of the spectrum was the fear, what if's, and anxiety. Dr. Mukta finally came in, after about twenty minutes, carrying a thick file and greeted us with pleasantries. As the words "Well, you don't have cancer!" rolled off her tongue, I let out a long sigh of relief. She went on to explain the results of my blood work and the other tests, and she said that they were all normal. She suggested I see a rheumatologist as she suspected inflammatory issues.

The stress of the last few weeks lifted, but the relief lasted for only a few moments until reality set in again. If it was not cancer, what was it? Right away, I felt as if I was back at square one. In those few moments, I felt complete discouragement because I knew the journey wasn't over and that the words Dr. Nancy had said, whatever it is, they will find it, weren't true. They didn't find it, and where did that leave me?

On the drive home, the question of where I would go from here kept circulating in my head. I felt like I'd exhausted all avenues, and there was nowhere else to turn. I had not seen my family doctor since his IBS diagnosis, and I didn't feel confident that if I went back to him, he could help me.

In retrospect, maybe he would have since my symptoms were now more than the stitch-like pain. I had lost the use of my arms, and my legs were also being affected, so maybe he would've pursued other possibilities. I couldn't bear the thought of him not supporting me, though, so I just didn't go back because I was so disappointed. Even if he ordered the same tests, I would've felt like I had somebody familiar in my corner, instead of seeing strangers who knew nothing about me, and the positive, upbeat person I was.

A few days later, Dr. Nancy called and said that the CT scan of my chest showed a mass on my right breast, and she wanted me to have a breast ultrasound and mammogram done. I think I was numb by this time and thought nothing of this. I wasn't scared or worried about what they might find because my experience so far had wreaked havoc on my emotional well-being. I tried to stay calm and positive because fighting depressive thoughts took more energy than I had. The mass turned out to be benign dense tissue in the breast—the end of another road.

Trying to get a family doctor in the town we lived in was impossible. We had tried for over nine years, ever since we moved from the city. Doctors were just not taking new patients. William happened to have a conversation with the dental hygienist who assisted Dr. Adam with my orthotic, and she said there was a new doctor in town who was taking new patients. I was especially excited because it was a female doctor. I thought that, maybe, she would be helpful regarding my menopausal symptoms, which had taken a back seat to everything else. My family doctor was over an hour's drive away, so we needed to find someone closer anyway. We waited for a month for the interview with the new doctor and mused that we would be interviewed, wondering about the possibility of us not being successful. It seemed a strange notion for a doctor to interview prospective patients, but I suppose we were also interviewing her.

We got to the meet and greet fifteen minutes early, to be polite, and were eager to meet a doctor with a fresh perspective. We waited for almost two hours in the biggest doctor's waiting room I'd ever seen. There was standing room only, with several people standing, and I wondered how long they had been waiting. We were finally called in and met first with the PA (Physician's Assistant), who explained how their system worked.

There was one doctor, Dr. Tatyana, and three PAs who saw patients. A PA could potentially see a patient at an appointment, but not more than twice. At the patient's third appointment, they would see the doctor. The system seemed quite an acceptable one, since sometimes one may just need to refill a prescription. We agreed that this would work for us, and the doctor came in. She was quite lovely and asked me about my medical history first and my most immediate issue that required assistance.

We went through my symptoms and the tests I'd had so far. Dr. Tatyana seemed quite keen and interested as we told her about my experience over the last fourteen months. When we told her about the tremors, and specifically when I got them, she looked at her assistant and said, "Sounds like the sympathetic and parasympathetic nervous systems."

Those words again! Tom, the physiotherapist, had explained about this nervous system before I heard Dr. Tatyana say the words a second time. The doctor rattled off a bunch of required tests to the PA, and by the end of the appointment, she ordered: A Holter Monitor, which I would wear for two weeks; an MRI of the brain; a pulmonary-function test; a sleep test; and blood work for lupus, among other things.

We told her that I already had a rheumatologist appointment booked for the end of July, and she thought it was an option to explore. Since nothing I took helped with pain, William insisted she prescribe something, and she prescribed pregabalin. I didn't want to get the drug because I didn't like the potential side effects, but I was so desperate that I decided to give it a try. We left the appointment with guarded hope that something would show up.

The first time I tried the pregabalin, I got extremely high and was zombie-like the next day, with no pain relief. We researched it and learned that it had to be used for some time for it to work. I took it for a week and finally gave up because it gave me additional symptoms of lethargy and tiredness. My lack of sleep by this point, because of the pounding and tremors, had taken its toll. The benefits of adding the side effects of this drug to the mix seemed minimal. William and I both had appointments for the sleep test at the end of June, and we joked that it would be our date night. I was also fitted with the heart monitor and wore this for two weeks. I asked the technician who set up the Holter Monitor if it was any different from the one I'd worn before because that one found nothing. He explained that, maybe, I needed to wear it for more than forty-eight hours.

I felt in my heart of hearts, no pun intended, that nothing was wrong with my heart per se, but that something else was wrong, and it was affecting how my heart worked. Who was I going to say this to without them looking at me like I had two heads since I had no medical background?

I didn't buy my family doctor's diagnosis of clogged arteries, primarily because I exercised and ate healthy, but more importantly, he had done no testing to confirm these alleged blockages. William researched menopausal symptoms, and heart-pounding and palpitations showed up as possible symptoms. The difference was my pounding was constant, 24/7, and it got worse if I did something as simple as walk up the stairs. My pounding wasn't fleeting or random, as suggested by the multiple sites we scoured. It was strange to me to have these symptoms, so explaining them to a doctor was daunting. I knew what I was feeling, but no amount of googling got me any closer to an explanation.

I wasn't sure about the sleep test either, even after the technician explained the process while hooking up what seemed like more than two dozen wires to my head and chest. He explained that the device recorded the number of times I awakened during the night. It also recorded my brain waves as I went through the various stages of sleep. I didn't put much weight on this test because I knew why I was waking up during the night. I was in so much pain, and when I turned, my body hurt more, and I woke right up. I also woke up when my heart pounded more than usual for no reason. Sometimes, it was a combination of the two—turning, which made my body hurt, which caused my heart to pound even more, after I was able to get past the tremors, which woke me when I was on the cusp of falling asleep. If nothing else, I thought the sleep test would prove that I was waking multiple times during the night, and maybe it would be enough to warrant further investigation.

We got the results of our sleep tests from the hospital, and mine confirmed that I did wake up many times during the night. "Time at lights out was 10:20 p.m. Latency to initial sleep onset was 32 minutes, and with minimal sleep during the first hour. A moderately fragmented sleep pattern was seen with 24 separate awakenings observed, and sleep efficiency reduced to 56%. Architecturally REM sleep was reduced to 9% total, and sleep stages were distributed otherwise as follows: Stage I: 6%, Stage II: 47%, Slow Wave: 38%."

The conclusion: "Severely fragmented sleep pattern with prolonged awakenings and reduced REM sleep" because of the "influence of foreign laboratory environment as well as an element of insomnia." I'm glad I didn't put too much weight on the results of this test, as it turned out nothing came of it. All this test proved was that I didn't have sleep apnea, which I believe was the goal in the first place. Since that was not an issue, the fact that I woke up twenty-four times from 10:20 p.m. to around 5:30 a.m. amounted to nothing. No one considered that I'd never had insomnia, or investigated the reason I woke up multiple times or had such a poor sleep pattern if it was not related to sleep apnea. The report stated that I had an acceptable subjective sleepiness score. *WHAT? I kept thinking, What a waste of resources!*

My blood work came back negative for lupus and other inflammatory diseases, and the only outstanding test from Dr. Tatyana was the MRI in September. By late July, the pain intensified, and I couldn't wait another two months for the MRI. I went to Dr. Tatyana's office after multiple attempts to get through to reception. The phone was on a constant loop, and when I chose the appropriate extension as prompted, it would say it was the wrong extension. Frustrated, tired, and in pain, I drove to the office and politely told the receptionist that something was wrong with their phone.

She very casually said, oh no, nothing is wrong. She didn't seem to be too concerned that calls were not getting through, and I didn't have it in me to deal with it. I asked if she could put me on a cancellation list for the MRI, and she said no, that I had to wait for the appointment. My next inquiry was about a clinic William had found in Buffalo, New York. I told her that we were willing to go there and pay $500 US to do the MRI, but we needed a referral from the doctor. I asked if I would be able to get one.

She said no and told me that the doctor was away on vacation, and the other PAs were busy. It just didn't seem to be my day. I asked if it were possible for her to call around to other testing clinics because we were willing to go wherever we could have it done sooner. Her response left me speechless for about fifteen seconds. She said, "You cannot access an MRI out of your local area, and you have to wait for the September appointment."

I then realized I was dealing with someone who didn't know her ass from her elbow. I politely said thank you and left, never to return to that doctor's office.

Oh, I was mad! Being mindful of all the signs posted about their zero-tolerance policy for abuse, aggression, and the like, I decided to make a speedy exit because I was about to lose control. I had been frustrated for so long, and I didn't want to take it out on this either unqualified or misinformed young lady. The idea that an administrative assistant working in a doctor's office thought a patient couldn't access health care outside of their county was ludicrous. I wrote a letter to Dr. Tatyana, outlining my reasons for not returning as a patient, and I am sure she never received it. Their model works very well in theory, but I couldn't understand why there was always an hour or more wait time when they had three PAs and the doctor seeing patients. I didn't have the time, patience, or ability to sit for such long periods in this doctor's office.

At my initial appointment with Dr. Tatyana, she had requested test results from my family doctor for the previous year, and I called his office to get the information sent. I found out that I had to pay a fee to transfer my file to a new family doctor. After some back and forth, the administrative assistant, Christy, was curious why I wanted to leave their office. I told her that the doctor diagnosed me with an illness I didn't have, and if she knew the hell I had been through over the last year, trying to find out what was wrong with me, she would understand.

I like Christy because she genuinely shows concern and empathy with patients. She proceeded to tell me that, if the doctor told me I had IBS, that's what I had because he was a very good doctor.

I felt like I was at the end of my rope! All I could do now was wait for whatever was causing such havoc in my life to paralyze me slowly. My limbs were locking up at an alarming rate, and I was losing my ability to use them more each day. At this point, I gave up. I had been running with my gaslight on for months, with little sleep and lots of frustration, and I mentally threw in the towel.

We went to the rheumatologist appointment at the end of July, as referred by the SOC Clinic. Even though I had pain in my arms and legs, I had no joint pain, but it was an option to explore. With every doctor I saw, I thought this is it—this would be the one to find out what was wrong with me.

Dr. Alan came into the office, and I couldn't believe how young he was! He was not the perceived image of a doctor wearing a white coat and glasses with a stethoscope around his neck! He wore skater shoes and a T-shirt that showed his belly when he raised his arms to show me how to raise my arms. We shared my medical history and symptoms, which by now, I was tired of reciting over and over, but I understood that it was part of the process. After he examined me, he said he would order musculoskeletal X-rays and blood inflammatory tests.

After asking me to do a few movements to see what I was capable of doing, we sat back at his desk to get his take on my symptoms. He slid a sheet of paper across the desk at us with an outline of the human body and asked me to write on it where my pain was. He then handed me some literature, and when I glanced at it, I got an awful feeling in my stomach.

He suggested that I look at the website listed on the brochure to find out more about fibromyalgia, since browsing the Internet was scary. (This was before I even had any of his tests done.)

William said, "Nah nah, she doesn't have fibromyalgia. That's not what it is," the frustration in his voice unmistakable. He told Dr. Alan that we just needed someone to go to bat for me, and I understood what he meant. Even though we'd had multiple tests done, and we were very grateful and appreciative of the doctors we'd seen up to that point, he wanted to feel as if there was one doctor in our corner, advocating for us. Dr. Alan responded quite hastily, "That's not me! My job is to find an autoimmune disease and kill her immune system with chemo!"

My eyes bulged out of my head in horror, and my jaw dropped! I could sense William's frustration turn to anger, and I immediately knew that it was time to get out of there. *Is this the new breed of doctors*? I mused. Was it even professional to say something of that nature to a patient who'd just explained her horrid experience so far? There was no empathy, or if he had any, he didn't show it. We thanked him for his time and left.

I did the X-rays and blood work on the same day in the same building, and the receptionist said she would send the results to Dr. Alan within two business days. Two days later, I called his office, and his receptionist said that they hadn't got the results. I asked her if there was a number where I could contact the radiologist's office, to ask about the results, and she said she didn't have a contact number, and that I had to wait. I waited another day and, thinking it didn't make sense that they didn't have a contact number for the office that they referred their patients to for X-rays, googled and got the phone number for the radiology office. I called, and the receptionist said that the results had been sent to the doctor's office at 4:20 p.m. on the same day.

I asked if she could send the results to my family doctor, and she agreed. I gave her the contact information and could hear her clicking away at her keyboard. About two minutes later, she said, "Done," meaning she had sent it successfully. Out of curiosity, I called the rheumatologist's office to find out whether they'd received the results, and I couldn't believe it when the receptionist told me they had still not received them. She also said that I would have to wait once they received them because Dr. Alan was away on vacation. I couldn't get over the apparent incompetence of the medical staff we encountered. Maybe I was just having the worst run of wrong timing that I'd ever had in my life. It didn't matter anyway, as we made a follow-up appointment to go back to my original family doctor.

The rheumatologist's report stated that my "symptoms appear to be in keeping with an inflammatory or rheumatological disorder. However, her blood work for these investigations up to date have been negative." It said that I had fourteen out of sixteen points for fibromyalgia, with a pain level of eleven out of twelve.

The pain had progressed so much now that I became dependent on William for everything. Even though he went with me to some of my appointments, I tried as much as possible to drive myself if one was close to home. I eventually gave up driving because I had no strength or mobility in my arms and couldn't move my neck. Sitting resulted in indescribable pain in my triceps, back, and my sides when leaning against anything. I also didn't feel safe driving because my cognitive skills had drastically declined from lack of sleep.

I was now running on empty. I could barely shower or get dressed on my own. By August, all I did was sit, even though sitting caused more pain as I leaned up against the sofa. There was no position I could find that gave some relief. It was evident to William that I had nothing left, and he took time off work to take care of me.

He decided to go back to our family doctor and insisted on an MRI of my head and stomach. He asked that I see an internal medicine specialist because of the stomach pains, which really hadn't moved but had increasingly gotten worse. He forcefully but respectfully told the doctor that I didn't have IBS since IBS doesn't cause the kind of symptoms I had.

Sensing William's anger, the doctor said he understood our frustration without offering much input on what other tests he thought I should have. Without question, he consented to William's requests for the MRIs. Christy was very efficient, getting the appointment for the MRI of my head within two days, although there was a catch: It was at 2:00 a.m., and we had to drive two and a half hours away. We certainly didn't mind because we were willing to go to Buffalo, which was further away if we were unable to get an earlier appointment.

Driving to the appointment and being up so late wreaked havoc on my body, but at least we didn't have to wait until September. By the following week, Christy arranged the MRI of my abdomen at a hospital that was not in the county in which we lived. I chuckled to myself when I thought of the receptionist who'd told me I couldn't, and I felt empathy for other patients who didn't know any better and who may have made a similar request.

We waited a few days for the results and returned yet again to my family doctor. The head non-contrast MRI: "No acute intracranial abnormality of space-occupying lesion detected... Notably, the distribution is not typical of MS."

It was a relief to rule this out, and maybe this is what Dr. Tatyana suspected when she'd ordered the MRI of my head. According to my family doctor, there was nothing remarkable in my test results from the rheumatologist, and no further testing was required. The end of another road!

I wish there were words to describe the frustration and discouragement I felt at this point. Even though I tried to look at it from the viewpoint that it was good that things were being ruled out, we still didn't know what was wrong, and I felt I was losing myself, bit by bit, every day.

In July, William insisted I see a chiropractor because of the lower back and neck pain, and I gave in after some hesitation. I was apprehensive of chiropractors because I was very uncomfortable with the idea of 'cracking' the spine. Two weeks before that dreaded day in late November of 2017, I had gone to a chiropractor on William's insistence, for pain in my mid-back on the left side. I saw him three times, and it was after my third adjustment, that I felt my jaw drop to the right. It moved as I could push it back to the left, and while doing so, it made a clicking sound but didn't stay. William pleaded with me to go and see another chiropractor, Dr. Mark, as he had the technology to do a spinal thermography, which would tell us about any issues of concern.

William took me to the appointment, and Dr. Mark did the scan and showed us what a normal scan of the spine looked like, and what the optimal nerve pattern should be, and compared it to mine. It showed that there were severe issues with my C1 vertebra, and mild and moderate issues with C3, C5, and L1, L3. His recommended care plan was two adjustments a week, with a full progress exam at six weeks.

We asked about the possibility of these adjustments, which I already knew I was not going to do, addressing the pain in my sides. We explained the squeezing, stitch like sensation in my stomach area, which got worse with movement. His response didn't convince me because I couldn't wrap my brain around the idea that spinal adjustments were going to alleviate my stomach pain, let alone the pain in my upper extremities. In the back of my mind, I was already aware of the time I'd 'wasted' with a dentist and physiotherapist, thinking their therapy would alleviate the stomach pains, so I didn't pursue treatments with Dr. Mark.

On our way back from seeing Dr. Mark, William called the radiology office and requested a copy of my X-rays. He wanted to look at the images himself, instead of taking the word of a radiologist. As soon as we got home, he inserted the disk into the computer with my X-ray images. When he saw the one of my C-spine, he exclaimed, "Something is wrong with your C-spine!"

He proceeded to show me the obvious problem, well obvious to him. William had a degree of medical knowledge, as he'd completed his B.Sc. at UCLA on a scholarship, as well as two years of medical school, before deciding to follow in his father's footsteps to start his own successful trucking company. He also has chiropractic adjustments regularly and has since he was five years old. He said that it was the thing to do before going back to school in September, as well as when hockey season was over. He insisted that we get a copy of the report from the rheumatologist, even though our doctor didn't say there was any reason for concern.

We got the report and scoured it, looking for anything out of the ordinary. Except for some mild degenerative changes of both hips, SI joints, and lumbosacral spine, and multi-level degenerative changes of the thoracic spine, everything was unremarkable.

The cervical spine also showed mild degenerative disease at C6/C7, with no significant narrowing identified on either side. According to the report, my features may be more in keeping with fibromyalgia, especially if malignant and inflammatory etiologies have been ruled out.

So, this was my diagnosis? Fibromyalgia? Even though my intuition told me I didn't have fibromyalgia, I was so mentally, emotionally, and physically exhausted that I said to William, "Maybe this is the issue, and now we just have to figure out how to treat it." At least my monster now had a name, and I could deal with it. He would not relent and insisted that I did not have fibromyalgia and to get it out of my head. We were awaiting the referral appointments for the internal medicine specialist as well as the neurologist. William kept telling me that we were getting closer to the real issue and to stop even thinking it was fibromyalgia because it wasn't.

My fiftieth birthday was about two weeks away. I'd never thought much about how I would celebrate this milestone year, but I certainly hadn't envisioned I would be waiting for yet another consultation with a doctor to figure out what was wrong. We met with the internal medicine specialist Dr. Fakh, and I immediately felt at ease with him. He reminded me of an old family friend who was a doctor when I was a young child.

He listened intently to my whole history of symptoms for over an hour and seemed quite empathetic to my plight. He examined my abdomen and didn't feel anything that caused him concern. He then proceeded to explain the findings on the MRI report, which indicated that both kidneys appeared normal, and images covering the liver, spleen, gall bladder, and pancreas appeared normal as well. No lymphadenopathy. Impression: Essentially, unremarkable study.

All of my organs were healthy. That was good to know, and it was a relief. But I couldn't help but feel like I wanted to scream from a hilltop, *"So what is causing my pain?! I'm not making this up! It is real, and it hurts!"*

My life had come to a complete stop, and I had to get help even to pull up my pants. Dr. Fakh saw how much pain I was in, and said to William that, if it got intolerable, he should take me to the hospital because "that's what hospitals are there for."

I'd already told William that, unless my insides were falling out, he was never to take me to a hospital again. I couldn't go through the ordeal of waiting in the ER for another thirteen or more hours. Even though I was in severe pain and felt hopeless and discouraged, the idea of going to a hospital again made me feel even worse.

The neurologist appointment followed not long after I saw Dr. Fakh, and when I heard his accent, I felt right at home. Dr. Andre and I were originally from the same country, and we shared a couple of stories about our previous lives there. We again gave him a rundown of my experience over the last fourteen months, my symptoms, and my experience with various tests, even though he could see it from my records. I was so tired of saying the same thing over and over again because it made me feel worse to relive it in words. William pointed out to him that he thought something was amiss with my nerves since I had a constant burning sensation on my skin on my arms and neck. After an examination, Dr. Andre confirmed that I had feeling in my extremities, so there was no cause for concern, and that there was nothing wrong with my nerves. William also pointed out that I had tingling in both hands, but it quickly became evident that nothing was going to come of this visit since I had sensation in my fingers, toes, and feet.

The cranial-nerve examination performed by the neurologist was unremarkable. His analysis indicated that I had mild weakness of the proximal upper extremities, with some give-way weakness secondary to pain involving the left shoulder... and of the left hip flexor. Overall, apart from brisk reflexes, which can sometimes suggest cervical spondylosis, her neurologic examination seems fairly benign. Sensory examination to pinprick and joint position sense was intact.

Dr. Andre said he would request a C-spine MRI and neuromuscular consultation, even though my nerves seemed healthy. I was appreciative, and we left, again, with a bit more hope that a diagnosis was just around the corner.

I had the EMG (electromyography) done on my fiftieth birthday! What a way to spend such a momentous day, but I couldn't postpone the appointment since thankfully, Dr. Andre had asked his colleague to expedite the test so that we wouldn't have to wait another few weeks.

The room with no windows was in the basement of the hospital, and it was small, cold, and dreary looking, with fluorescent lighting. We went through the entire story yet again with this doctor, reliving the whole ordeal in words. William brought the thermography scan done by Dr. Mark and asked the specialist if he would look at it, as it might help.

He answered quite quickly: "I don't know anything about that." His response took me a bit by surprise. Maybe he noticed our reaction and said he would look at it after he completed his EMG. William was sure that this would reveal the issue, as he insisted that the tingling in my fingers, and burning in my neck and arms indicated something was wrong with my spine, which he believed affected my nerves.

I changed into the hospital gown with William's assistance. I got on the examination table, going over the last year and four months in my head, wondering how much longer and how many more doctor visits I would have to endure. Dr. Al-Noor stuck pins into my toes and fingers and left arm and sent a wave of electricity through them. As if the pain I was in wasn't already bad enough, this certainly didn't make it better.

The sensation of the electric pulse going into my skin exaggerated the pain I already had and probably felt worse than it was. My attempts to hold back the tears failed miserably, and the doctor apologized and assured me it would be over soon. After what seemed like forever, it was finally over, and he asked me to get dressed. I was happy we didn't have to wait weeks for these results, as he would have them right away. We sat down with the doctor, ready to hear the results, full of anticipation and confidence that this test would reveal the name of my monster.

"I have good news and bad news," said Dr. Al-Noor.

I never really liked the good news, bad news game, because if you got the bad news first, it spoiled the following good news, and if you got the good news first, the bad news spoiled it.

"There is nothing wrong with you" was the good news, and "I don't know what's causing your pain" was the bad news. The report from Dr. Al-Noor (MD FRCP) stated: There is no significant neuromuscular abnormality on today's examination. There is no significant evidence of peripheral neuropathy, peripheral nerve entrapment, myopathy, or myositis.

Our hopes dashed once again! This time I was too numb to feel much. I was tired and drained and wanted to forget everything for the rest of the day and just enjoy my birthday. My problems would be there tomorrow to deal with, and I wanted to salvage my day, knowing that, for as long as I lived, I would always remember what I had done on the day I turned fifty.

Kathryn had invited us for lunch, and we enjoyed one of my favorite dishes: South Indian food and for dessert, her famous double-fudge chocolate cake, which I relished. I tried to be as upbeat as I could under the circumstances and enjoyed the rest of my special day.

I didn't think a body could be in so much pain twenty-four hours a day, seven days a week! I felt stuck in a cycle of pain and sleeplessness. It was difficult to fall asleep because of the tremors, and if/when I was able to doze off, the pain woke me. If my body was attempting to heal in any way, the lack of sleep prevented that, as the body heals when it's at rest.

Four days after my birthday, I had the MRI of my C-spine. As I waited for the procedure to begin, I had a sense of déjà vu, as I had been here just a few weeks earlier. The technician was friendly and had a dry sense of humor and made me laugh for a few minutes with his antics. He gave me instructions and explained what I would hear and feel so that I would be comfortable with the procedure. Because this was my third MRI, I was quite familiar with the loud sounds the machine made during the process. It didn't take very long, and we went home again with renewed hope that this test would find my issue.

William looked again at the X-rays of my C-spine and insisted the problem stemmed from there. The question was why I had the stitch like pains in my sides if the problem stemmed from my C-spine. Neither of us could answer this, but we were sure the MRI would clear things up.

Two days later, I awoke from a night of little sleep and lots of tears, for the pain seemed to get worse by the minute. I told William that, even though I wanted to avoid going to any hospital with every fiber of my being, I needed to go to the hospital because the pain was excruciating. The words of Dr. Fakh swirled in my head: That's what hospitals are there for! I couldn't take it anymore, and my even asking to go to the hospital spoke volumes about the level of my pain. Our follow-up appointment with Dr. Andre wasn't until September seventh because he was on vacation, and the thought of waiting for more than a week with this pain was too much to bear. We didn't miss anything by not seeing him about the MRI results, because his report said the following:

MRI C-SPINE:

INDICATION: 49-year-old female with weakness and hyperreflexia.

COMPARISON: No prior images available for comparison.

TECHNIQUE: Multisequence multiplanar MRI images through the cervical spine without contrast administration.

FINDINGS:

There is normal alignment of the cervical spine.

Vertebral body heights are preserved. Vertebral signal is unremarkable. No evidence of recent or remote fracture of the vertebral bodies.

The spinal cord is of normal signal and caliber.

The craniocervical junction is unremarkable in appearance.

Assessment of the central canal and neural foramina are as follows:

C2/C3: No significant central canal or foraminal stenosis.

C3/C4: There is a small disc osteochondral bar. No significant central canal narrowing. No significant foraminal stenosis.

C4/C5: No significant central canal or foraminal stenosis.

C5/C6: No significant central canal or foraminal stenosis.

C6/C7: There is a small broad-based disc osteochondral bar. The central canal demonstrates mild narrowing. There is mild right foraminal narrowing. The left neural foramen is not significantly narrowed.

C7/T1: No significant central canal or foraminal stenosis.

Limited views of the intracranial structures demonstrate no significant abnormality.

No notable soft tissue abnormality is seen.

OPINION:

PAGE 1   Signed Report Printed From PCI   (CONTINUED)

I knew when he did his exam in his office that it would be a waste of time to go back to him. I realized he didn't seem to grasp the severity of my condition when he commented on my mild pain.

William called the hospital, where I did the MRI to find out if the results were ready. They were, so we got in the car for the hour-and-fifteen-minute drive, which seemed so much longer to me. He got a copy of my MRI on a CD, and we headed downtown to St. Michael's Hospital. We drove into the ambulance area of the ER because I couldn't walk from the parking area back to the hospital. William went in and told the nurse that I couldn't walk, and they sent someone out with a wheelchair.

I could barely lift my arms, and my legs hurt to walk. I felt as though, whatever was wrong with me, I was fighting a losing battle. I dreaded the long wait time in the ER and even being in this kind of environment. William parked the car, came back, and never left my side, reassuring me that everything would be fine and that if anyone could find out what was wrong, the doctors at St. Michael's would.

He'd had prior experience with the doctors here and was confident that this would be our last stop. We went through the typical registration process, and the staff was patient and accommodating. We had to wait until we were called, like everybody else who was not an urgent case. They called us about forty-five minutes later, and I was surprised and comforted myself with the thought that maybe this wouldn't be as bad as I'd imagined.

We waited another hour or so until we saw a nurse who did the intake, and we again related the history of my symptoms. William told him we had a copy of my C-spine MRI on a CD, along with all other reports from day one of my ordeal. We thought it would save time and resources because I already had done all the tests, so they wouldn't have to do them again. Besides, we just wanted someone to give us feedback regarding the C-spine MRI. The nurse said that they would do their blood work, in case other testing missed something. We were then sent to another, more private room, which I appreciated, because there was an examination table and I could stretch out, since sitting for so long aggravated my pain. The on-call ER doctor showed up and retook a history of my symptoms. His shift would be over soon, and we didn't see him again.

More time went by, and a young intern came in and asked me to tell my story again. I did, and he said his colleague would be by to talk with us. We waited for what seemed like two hours before another young intern came by and asked us to tell her about my symptoms again. She listened very attentively as they all did, and I tried to be as specific and detailed as possible because I thought maybe she would pick up on something that the other doctors may have missed along the way.

She asked a couple of questions, which I answered. Then I asked her if I could ask a question. She said yes, and I asked if she'd ever heard of the kind of tremors I had been experiencing and gave her a synopsis of what they felt like and when I got them. I got the feeling she thought I was bizarre when she said she'd never heard about tremors such as these. I told her about the pain at the back of my head, which felt like a squeezing sensation. I described the pain that ran from the back of my head to the skin in my outer ears, especially the left one. She didn't take any notes, and I couldn't help but wonder how she would remember everything I told her, because it was a lot. She said they were very busy and she would be back and left the room.

We waited another couple of hours. I could barely find a comfortable position that didn't cause intolerable pain. The pain felt like a hot rod ran into the base of my skull and intensified when I rested my head on a surface. The nurse told us that pillows were a hot commodity in the hospital, so there were none. After about four hours of getting to the hospital, the nurse who did the intake came and said that he would admit me, and someone would be by to take me to a room.

Everyone we dealt with was very professional and made me feel comfortable, and I kept thinking, *this is it. Someone here will finally figure it out, and my ordeal will soon end.* The nurse got me a sandwich, which I ravenously ate since we'd been there for about six hours. William refused to leave me when I told him to go out and get something to eat because he wanted to be there when the doctor came by. We got to the hospital in the early afternoon, and it was close to midnight when they moved me to a room not too far from where we originally were. William helped me to get cleaned up for bed, and a few minutes after I settled in for the night, they said I would be transferred to another room.

I tried to stay positive, especially after the nurse said that we would see a team of specialists the next morning. I would have been quite happy just seeing a neurologist, but a team sounded more promising. I was put in a private room, quite different from a typical hospital room as it was glass all around, and given a sedative and pain meds. I didn't know what they were but took them anyway, desperate for relief.

The bed wasn't a typical hospital bed either, more like an examination table, and it was not comfortable because it was so narrow. I was in this room maybe forty-five minutes before another nurse came and said I had to move again, this time to a standard hospital room I shared with another patient. The sedative didn't work, and I was still up at 2:00 a.m. William asked the nurse if there was something else she could give to help me get to sleep, and she brought me yet another sedative.

The female intern who saw us in the ER came by and asked how I was doing. When William told her about my pain, she asked if she should give me intravenous pain meds. He said no, though, because nothing seemed to work. William stayed at my bedside the whole time, and I think I finally dozed off around 4:00 a.m. The pain didn't let me sleep for very long, as usual, and I awoke feeling a bit disoriented, not remembering where I was for a few seconds. William wasn't where I'd last seen him, in a chair next to the bed, and I became a bit frantic and called the nurse. She told me that he had gone out to the car, and so I called him on his cell phone. He got back to the room quickly and said that he was tired and couldn't sleep in the chair, so when I finally fell asleep, he'd gone to the car and was able to get an hour or so. He told me that he watched me as I slept, and I woke up every ten to twelve minutes, groaned in pain, and then dozed back off to sleep.

We knew the team of doctors would make their rounds around 10:00 a.m., so I got ready and waited for their arrival. The attending doctor, Dr. James, came by and said that we would have more privacy if we went to a nearby conference room. I sensed William's eagerness at the mere thought of laying it all out on the table because he believed with all his heart that my problems stemmed from my spine. He wheeled me into the dimly lit conference room. There were about five, maybe six other very young people already seated at the table. Dr. James asked if it was okay that they were there, and I agreed and wondered if this was the team of specialists. He said that they were interns, and I speculated about how much experience they had, but I told myself to keep an open mind.

William couldn't wait to get to the whiteboard to draw it all out for them, but this didn't happen, as the meeting took a completely different turn than the one we anticipated.

The female intern who had listened to my history of symptoms in the ER the previous night read from her notes everything I told her, practically word for word. It was very detailed, just as I'd described. It impressed me that she'd remembered so much because she didn't take notes during our conversation. It was as if she recorded our conversation because her recollection of my symptoms was quite extraordinary. Especially, I thought, having worked (I'm sure) a twelve-hour or more shift, seeing various patients with various symptoms. When the intern finished, Dr. James, who sat crossed-legged with a notepad on his lap, scribbling as he listened to the intern, raised his head. His glasses were poised at the end of his nose as he looked over them at William and me, and asked if we agreed with everything the intern had read. We said that, yes, we agreed.

After telling us that I'd had a plethora of tests done as well as the blood work they did the night before, which were negative for any disease, he said, "There is nothing wrong with you!"

I was in total shock, and my eyes filled with tears, and my heart raced. I kept my composure when I felt a wave of heat move over my body. The thought ran through my head: *If a doctor at such a reputable hospital said nothing was wrong with me, then this indeed was the end of the road.*

After talking a bit more about all the tests I had, which showed nothing, he looked at William, wagged his index finger at him, and said, "It's time to get your wife off the medical treadmill and stop taking her from doctor to doctor."

If hearing the words nothing is wrong with you didn't cut like a knife, this statement was full of implications, the most important being that I shouldn't or couldn't seek any further medical investigations. I knew in my heart that I would end up immobile.

I didn't think I could've felt any worse, but then he continued on his verbal tirade: "Some people would kill for your results." He then proceeded to tell a story about a patient who came to the ER with headaches, and they couldn't find anything wrong with her after she had various tests.

He said, "She had gone up north to a mental health retreat and was cured."

I could see the steam coming out of William's ears, and he then interjected. "So let me ask you something: The body doesn't send a signal to the brain that you have pain unless you have pain?"

The doctor responded. "Oh, yes, it does!"

"Do tell," William said.

Dr. James explained that whatever was happening with me was a mind-body thing that they didn't understand and wasn't within their medical scope.

I could hear the disgust in William's tone. He then turned to the young interns, and said, "Let me ask you a question. If a patient comes to you presenting with signs of a pinched sciatic nerve, what are their symptoms? It's a burning, shooting, stabbing, throbbing pain coming out of their ass, and it's either going down their right leg or their left leg. Would you agree?"

All the interns nodded their heads in agreement.

William said, "Exactly! My wife has the same problem, but it's coming out of her neck."

None of them responded verbally, but Dr. James kept on his dialogue about the mind-body connection being something that is not fully understood. At this point, I spoke up, saying that I was quite aware of the mind-body connection because I was a Reiki Master, and I was quite mindful of the possibility of thoughts affecting one's health. I told them that, because I understand the mind-body connection, I had seen a psychotherapist.

"Did you pay for this service?" asked Dr. James

"Yes," William said, "a hundred dollars an hour." His response was even more confusing and disturbing.

"Oh, he's not a real doctor!"

I didn't know if I should laugh or cry, and I thought I could've saved myself $700. What kind of doctor did I pour my heart out to, if Philip wasn't a real doctor?

I wanted Dr. James and the interns to understand that, even if they didn't understand the mind-body connection, I understood it. I told them that it had been scientifically proven, for example, that being around a body of water has a calming effect on the mind, which results in physiological changes in the body, and that the phenomenon is known as blue mind.

I said research showed that simply being near the waters' edge affected the mental state of a person. In the experiment, the participants' heart and pulse rates were reduced, which resulted in a calmer state. I talked briefly about the effects of meditation on the mind, and about being in nature, for example, walking on grass and its grounding effects. There was one male intern in the room, and in my peripheral vision, I noticed he nodded his head, and I thought he agreed with me. The other interns watched me with blank stares on their faces, and no one said anything.

I thought that, just maybe, there was one person who did understand the mind-body connection, and I said to him, "You're nodding your head yes. Do you understand what I'm saying?"

He then looked like a deer caught in headlights, his eyes opened wide and a confused expression on his face. He quickly shook his head to indicate he didn't understand. I thought to myself, *if these are the kind of doctors medical schools are producing, we are in big trouble!* And worse, that Dr. James was training them to view patients the same way he does.

I wanted to get out of the conference room, hospital, and city as fast as I could because I couldn't bear to listen to any more of Dr. James' reprimands that I was making up this pain in my head. The combination of anger, fear, resentment, frustration, and pure disbelief over what had transpired left me emotionally drained. The words to describe how I felt about this doctor and the interns in the room who tried to convince me that my pain was not real, don't exist. (Actually, the words do exist, but I'm trying to keep the party polite.)

We went back to the room, and the nurse told us that we had to wait for the doctor to discharge me. We waited for almost an hour until one of the interns who was in the meeting room came by and handed me a single sheet of paper. I looked at it and read the following:

I came to the hospital on August 29, 2018, and left on August 30, 2018.
I came in because of Somatoform Disorder.

I didn't know what the term somatoform meant, but the word disorder gave me a chill when I read it. I asked for clarification because no one used the word disorder in the conference room. I don't remember what the intern said, but she pointed to the information on the page regarding follow-up, medications, and rationale. The doctor prescribed: lorazepam for insomnia and anxiety and baclofen for muscle rigidity and tightness.

We took the envelope, thick with all of my test results from the last sixteen months, and left the hospital. I don't remember much of the drive home because I was so exhausted from the lack of sleep and the emotional roller coaster from my experience over the last, almost twenty-four hours. The words of Dr. James kept echoing in my ears, that I was making up pain because nothing was physically wrong with me. After we got home and I got settled, I decided to seek the knowledge of my friend Google to find out what somatoform disorder was.

> Somatoform disorders are a group of psychological disorders in which a patient experiences physical symptoms that are inconsistent with or cannot be fully explained by any underlying general medical or neurologic condition. Medically unexplained physical symptoms account for as many as 50% of new medical outpatient visits.[6]

FIFTY PERCENT! The idea that 50 percent of people seeking medical attention in an ER have a mental illness was mind-boggling to me. I was now part of this statistic, and I knew something was wrong in my body. My pain was real, and there was a reason for it! The article went on to talk about healthy children who express emotional distress in terms of physical pain. This information didn't seem relevant to me, so I checked the next hit. I read that "somatic symptom disorder (SSD, formerly known as somatization disorder or somatoform disorder) is a form of mental illness that causes one or more bodily symptoms, including pain. The symptoms may or may not be traceable to a physical cause."[7]

The words mental illness burned holes in my eyes! The doctor said that it was all in my head in the conference room, but never in a million years had I thought I would have an official mental illness diagnosis! Dr.

James didn't indicate to us that he, or any of the interns in the room, had any sort of training in psychology, psychotherapy, or psychiatry, or were qualified to diagnose me with a mental illness.

The only two interns who'd spoken were the ones who read my symptoms and the male intern, who only nodded, no. So I am not sure who came up with the diagnosis. I wasn't sure what to feel: despair, anger, or pessimism! I think I felt all of them, and the next few weeks, things went downhill really fast. I started to question my sanity and thought that maybe I was making it up in my head because I had all the possible tests, and there seemed no valid reason for my pain.

After all, doctors know how the human body works, and if they couldn't find anything wrong with me, maybe I was making it up. Perhaps I should seek out the mental health retreat up north to see if I could figure out my mental health issue! Maybe I needed to seek the help of a real doctor since, according to Dr. James, the one we paid for wasn't real. Something in my gut kept saying this was not right, though, and I had to stop thinking this way because I did not have a mental illness.

My made-up pain and symptoms eventually got so bad that I slept less and less. I had trouble getting to sleep because of the tremors, and if I managed to because of sheer exhaustion, I was awakened by the pounding or the pain in my arms, neck, sides, or head. The pounding also intensified as I cried and turned in the bed, and the anxiety, pain, and frustration resulted in hours of weeping.

In June, one of William's co-workers overheard him when another colleague asked how I was. She'd heard about our ordeal trying to find out what was wrong with me, the misdiagnoses as far as he was concerned, and the severe pain I had. She mentioned that, through his insurance coverage at work, we had access to a program that was a diagnostic and treatment support service. According to the brochure, the service allows access to the expertise of specialists, resources, information, and clinical guidance … by drawing on a global database of up to fifty thousand peer-ranked specialists.

We didn't have a diagnosis, not a relevant one anyway, so we thought we had nothing to lose. William went through the grueling process of providing the caseworker with information, recent health records, reports, and filling out pain questionnaires. I had become an observer at this point, as having this conversation caused me even more anxiety.

When I read the correspondence about the fifty thousand peer-ranked specialists, I thought for sure that someone would pick up on something that all the other doctors so far had missed. For two months, we went back and forth with the nurse practitioner in charge of my case, and I e-mailed her several updates about my worsening symptoms in great detail. I told her my pain had gotten so bad that I finally caved and went to the hospital and sent her a report of my experience.

In my last communication with the nurse, I told her that it would be my last e-mail, as it had become too painful to type. We waited for the report from this organization because we envisioned a team of specialists (not like the supposed one we'd met with at St. Michael's) around a table, not only reading the radiologists' reports but looking at my X-rays and MRIs, especially that of my C-spine.

A few days later, I got an e-mail with an attached report from the doctor who handled my case: the Director of Education & Fellowship Training, Associate Professor of Medicine at Harvard Medical School. My eyes couldn't move fast enough down the page as the report regurgitated all of my previous test results.

According to the medical report, "the possibility of a somatoform disorder is also possible. These two conditions share many features. Both conditions can develop insidiously, as was the case for our patient. These pain syndromes all develop due to a disorder of pain regulation called central sensitization that results in the pain signals being amplified in the brain centers that regulate pain. The pain felt in one part of the body may trigger pain sensitizations in other areas and explains why these conditions can be baffling."

The report was thirty-one pages long, and after I read that part, I stopped. Something in me shifted, and I knew this doctor was wrong. As William says, when he knows he is right about something, I thought this doctor could go pound sand up his a$$. Even though I almost believed the somatoform-disorder diagnosis, it was a load of poppycock. (I am being nice by using that word to describe what I thought of the report.) My mental decline had continued fast the few days after we got back from the hospital, but something happened when I read this diagnosis that lit a fire in me.

William continuously cautioned me, daily, not to believe the doctors, as he knew in his gut, that none of their diagnoses was correct. He was sure something was wrong with my spine. Part of me was hopeful, but the other part questioned where to go from there. There was no one else to turn to for help because we'd exhausted all our resources.

In July, William took me to a naturopathic doctor, Dr. Michelle, who specialized in women's issues for my menopausal symptoms. The hot flashes and what I call terror attacks exacerbated an already complicated problem, both physically and mentally. Dealing with pain 24/7 was dreadful, but additional emotional symptoms like mood swings, bouts of depression, and the terrible feeling of anxiety and terror, even though it only lasted the few seconds preceding a hot flash, were unbearable. I told myself that it would only be for a few moments and to breathe through it, but the feeling when it happened was absolute panic, and at the moment it happened, I didn't remember what it was. I didn't want to go on regular hormone-replacement therapy because I'd been on the pill for so long and didn't wish to put more synthetic hormones in my body. Dr. Michelle was very supportive as she listened to our story for over an hour. In her practice, she'd heard many unusual stories, so mine was not alarming by any means. But she had no clue what was causing my pain.

When we told her of the somatoform-disorder diagnosis, her eyes just about popped out of her head, and she was livid. She was very animated and seemed passionate about her work and discounted the diagnosis. She enthusiastically took notes, and at the end of the retelling of our story, she turned to me and said, "Do you know what your problem is?"

Part of me got excited for the few seconds it took to respond, "No. What?"

She looked right at me and said, "Your problem is that you don't look sick!" She said that I looked like nothing was wrong with me, and that was a problem. I understood that she meant that anyone looking at me would think nothing was wrong with me if I described my symptoms to them.

I said, "Well, I don't know how to look sick!" I assume this is why doctors like those at St. Michael's didn't believe something was medically wrong with me. I didn't look sick!

She ordered tests to confirm that I was menopausal because, according to my family doctor, I wasn't.

I didn't need a test to tell me that I was menopausal, but the results confirmed it. Dr. Michelle prescribed bioidentical progesterone, estrogen, and estriol, and the treatment helped with some of the menopausal symptoms. She thought the progesterone would help with the sleeping issues, and when it didn't, she suggested that I double up on the dose. That didn't help either because I didn't have trouble falling asleep but for the tremors.

She also didn't know what was causing the tremors as she'd never heard of this symptom before. William had researched it online, trying to see if anyone out in the stratosphere experienced this seemingly strange symptom. He happened onto a menopausal blog, where women described having the same tests I had to figure out what caused their tremors. When their doctors determined nothing was wrong, they too were prescribed antianxiety drugs.

The common thread running through these women's experiences was they were all premenopausal or menopausal. William shared the link with Dr. Michelle, and we thought we had figured out at least one of my so-far inexplicable symptoms. What made my tremors different was that theirs came on during the day: if they were watching TV or reading in bed. My tremors only came on as I was dozing off to sleep, and this difference showed that, even though I had other menopausal symptoms, my tremors probably weren't menopause related.

Dr. Michelle asked us to keep her apprised on how we were progressing with our investigation, and William kept in contact with her and shared the results from Harvard Medical when we got them. She just about blew a gasket when he told her what the doctor's diagnoses were. She agreed that they were wrong and told William to continue on the search because we would find out what the real issue was. I was so out of it that all I could do was sit and listen to his phone conversations.

William told anyone who would listen about my plight and our efforts for figuring out what was causing my physical decline. Of course, somebody always knows someone who may be able to help. Genaro, William's friend who put us in touch with the weed guy, invited him to a barbecue. Genaro's wife asked William how I was because Genaro had shared our story with her. He gave her an update of my condition so far, and she mentioned that there was a lady in town who, through a blood analysis, could tell someone what disease they had. He told me this when he returned home that night, and I thought it sounded too good to be true because if this were even the slightest bit possible, we wouldn't need doctors. Out of pure desperation, we went to this lady and experienced a comedy of errors that was quite entertaining.

After she asked us a little about my experience, she took a sample of my blood, put it on her slide, and was utterly bewildered why the image on her monitor screen was blurred. William kicked me under the table, and I looked over and saw him trying not to laugh. He told her it was because the lens was dirty. She insisted it wasn't and tried a few times to get a clear picture of my blood sample. William kicked me again, and I kicked him back to say stop because now I wanted to laugh. After a few minutes of messing around with the thing, she finally listened to him and used a clean lens and was surprised when a clear image of my cells appeared on her monitor, after trying another blood sample.

After considering the image for a few seconds, she walked over to a chart that hung on the wall, with different pictures of blood cells and explanations of what they meant. He kicked me again under the table, and I tried to ignore him because I was thinking the same thing he was: This lady said she'd worked with a naturopath who taught her this procedure and that she had been doing it for over ten years, and she still had to consult with a chart?!

My diagnosis ranged from absurd to downright incorrect. First off, I had a lot of blood cells dying. Kick. A spleen-related condition. Kick. My lymph system was sluggish. Kick. My body was riddled with candida and inflammation. Kick. It was also possible that I had a leaky gut, necrotic tissue, and my blood cells looked like a smoker's.

She recommended a couple of herbal remedies for my varying conditions and gave us a coupon for a health-food store. We thanked her, paid the $130 for this complete waste of our time, and laughed all the way home. On the receipt she gave us, it stated that our visit was for an initial nutritional analysis.

I was thankful for the comic relief because it had been a long time since I'd laughed, and even though my situation was serious, her analysis was so ridiculous that laughter was the only way to deal with it. I am sure that she was of help to someone, but I was not one of the lucky ones.

THE DIAGNOSIS IS IN
THE DETAILS

When we got home from the hospital, William inserted the CD with the image of my C-spine MRI into the laptop, and as soon as it appeared on the screen, he blurted out, "See, I told you so! Something is wrong with your spine." He pointed out C6/C7, and I was shocked when it became clear that something was wrong here. With my nonexistent knowledge of reading and interpreting MRIs, I said to him that the report, which we got from our family doctor, stated that there was indeed an issue where he suspected it was, but that it was unremarkable.

He wouldn't relent and insisted we see a chiropractor. As I heard the word again, I cringed. I didn't want to go to another chiropractor because the idea of someone cracking anything on me made me hurt more. He called Dr. Michelle and asked if she could recommend a good chiropractor, and she gave him a couple of referrals. Over the next few days, he spoke with both chiropractors to figure out what techniques they used, and if they had methods other than manual manipulation. I listened to him as he asked specific questions, and he finally decided on the one for which Dr. Michelle had a preference.

William made an appointment with Dr. Aron, and on September fourth, we had our first consultation. I wasn't sure about any of this, but I didn't have the energy to say otherwise. I went to the appointment without much hope of anything, since I couldn't bear to hear yet again that nothing was wrong with me.

William insisted there was a problem in my spine, and he was sure a chiropractor would see it. We took the X-rays and MRI with us, in case I needed to do X-rays, we wouldn't have to go through the process again. I felt like I was running out of time, and a few days could have made a difference in me giving up, unable to get out of bed because of the pain and because the muscles in my arms and legs felt so tight.

Dr. Aron was a personable doctor, and we gave him a rundown of my experience so far. He looked at my X-rays on his computer and proceeded to define the kind of pain I had in my sides. With his right hand, he pulled the left side of his T-shirt toward his right side and said my sides felt as if they were twisted. I couldn't believe my ears! Without me describing my pain as the squeezing-pulling sensation, here was someone who knew what I had been feeling for over seventeen months.

In those few moments following Dr. Aron's description of my pain, there was such relief that someone knew my pain was real and that I wasn't making it up in my head. It was even more surprising that I didn't have to tell him what I felt because he knew without my having to explain it.

I asked Dr. Aron what was wrong, and quite casually, he said I had "upper cervical subluxation complex."

"That's a mouthful," I said, having never heard the word subluxation before. "What does that mean?"

He explained that C1, the first vertebra of my spine (which is also called the atlas), had rotated. He compared what happened to a golf ball sitting on its tee, which sort of tilted off to the side. My nerves, tendons, muscles, and fascia moved along with the shifted vertebrae (issue at C1 affects C2). He explained I also had an issue (the chiropractic term is subluxation) at C6/C7, which was responsible for the pain in my neck, arms, and fingers.

I saw pure relief in William's face as he realized he'd been right all along. For me, it was a mixture of relief, hope, and anger. Relief now that my monster had a name, hope for the future because I could deal with it, and anger because I'd had to endure so much to get to this point, with no new information.

Dr. Aron shared his experience with a C-spine injury and the technique he'd developed because of it. He was driving and was hit from behind by another vehicle. Because he turned his head to the right at the time of impact, what might have been a simple case of whiplash, became a more severe injury, resulting in the same kind of symptoms I had.

"But what about the pain in my sides?" I asked because it didn't make sense to me that an issue in my neck could cause such terrible squeezing sensations in and around my last set of ribs.

He explained that nerves and muscles that come out of the C-spine connect to nerves and muscles in my sides, and that is why I had the stitchy pulling sensation. As he talked, the information swirled around in my head. Logically, it made sense, but I still had so many questions. Since this was our first one-hour consultation, there wasn't much time to ask all the questions I wanted to ask. He took photos from my shoulders up, and when he showed them to me, I couldn't believe it was me. My head looked as if someone photoshopped it onto my neck, and it looked one-sided and pushed forward. I'd never really noticed this, but I remember William telling me a year or so before that I needed to stand straight up, tits out because my posture was forward-leaning. He said this to me even before I had any symptomatic pain.

In his report, Dr. Aron said my prognosis for pain/symptom reduction, postural improvement, range of motion/movement, and improved strength was excellent. His work was to remodel and restructure the upper cervical spine, associated muscles, and connective tissue. Decompress and relieve pressure to irritated nerves. Reprogram problematic postural patterns, movement, and spinal deviations. Relieve pressure and tension in the skull and associated tissue.

Frequency of care was twice a week for four to six weeks, and he would work with me for an hour at $300 an hour. Our insurance benefits by this time had run out because I'd had physiotherapy and chiropractic care, so we paid out of pocket for my treatment. I thought his fee was steep, but since he had a customized technique, it seemed worth it. William and I shared my apprehension with Dr. Aron regarding the manual cracking of anything, and he assured me that his method didn't involve manual manipulation of the spine, as he worked specifically with the tissue. I said that this was the only way I would agree to treatment. I felt comfortable that he understood my experience and pain, but I couldn't help but wonder why this had happened to my spine, because I didn't have an injury.

When I got home, I googled the word subluxation and scoured the many hits that came up. The medical definition is "a partial dislocation of a joint. A complete dislocation is a luxation."[8] I also learned that, according to the WHO (World Health Organization), "it is a significant structural displacement. Therefore unlike the chiropractic belief of vertebral subluxation, it is always visible on static imaging studies such as X-rays."[9]

What?! I thought, *Unlike*!? It was visible on my X-rays and C-spine MRI, but according to the radiologists and medical doctors, it was unremarkable. It was because William looked at the images and didn't depend solely on the radiologists' reports, that he saw the issues and knew that what it showed was remarkable for me. I wanted to explore it even further and found videos on YouTube. The first hit when I searched atlas subluxation was a video by Dr. Mandell, explaining a bit more about what Dr. Aron talked about, and it made all the sense in the world. I was way beyond any self-help though, as my arms had locked up, and I couldn't raise them higher than a few inches from my sides.

On September 6, 2018, I had my first treatment with Dr. Aron while William walked around town. I asked how he was going to get my vertebrae back to how they should be. I couldn't comprehend how this had even happened to me and wanted to understand everything there was to know about my 'injury.' He explained it like this:

Imagine there is a pole (my spine) with multiple ropes (tissue, nerves, muscles) coming out of it, going in different directions. The problem is that the pole is not straight, but it should be. It then causes the ropes to strain at various points, which is why I felt the tight, twisting sensation in my body. For the pole to straighten, the attached ropes had to be manipulated, but it would take time. After all the time trying to figure out what was wrong, somebody finally gave an explanation, which logically seemed to make sense.

I felt comfortable that I was on the right track and looked ahead to being well again. When I had my first treatment, I didn't expect the kind of pain I experienced. Dr. Aron stretched and manipulated the tissue and muscles in my back, neck, and arms, and there were times I didn't think I would make it to the end of the hour. The pain was so excruciating, and I tried all I could to hold back the tears (and cuss words). I knew there was no other way to get healthy again, so I made up my mind to endure the pain.

For months, I hadn't moved my arms and neck, and the connective tissue (fascia) had, in effect, froze where it was. The tissue had to be broken up, and the stretching and manipulation would accomplish this.

After my sessions, William had to help me walk and lift my legs when I got in the car because they were so weak and painful. When we got home after my first treatment, I couldn't hold back the tears and cried so uncontrollably that he got scared and called Dr. Aron. He told him that my pain seemed worse than before, and he was concerned something else was wrong. Dr. Aron assured him that the pain I was experiencing was normal and part of the healing process because I was now moving muscles, ligaments, and so on, that had been dormant for so long.

Sometimes during the sessions, it seemed like I felt better. As painful as it was when the doctor manipulated and stretched my muscles, I was able to move my arms a bit better, but the pain was still intolerable. I think I convinced myself that the treatments were working because I knew the importance of a positive state of mind as it affects one's ability to heal.

At one of my treatments, I sat in a chair as the doctor worked on my neck from behind. He placed one hand under my chin and the other on top of my head. Without warning, he quickly turned my head and cracked my neck. His manual cracking of my neck caught me by surprise, and even though it didn't cause much additional pain at the time, this was not our deal. He was not supposed to crack anything on me, and I was not happy he did this. Even though I didn't feel any worse, I didn't feel any better either, and I said to him that he'd said he wouldn't manually crack my neck. He didn't seem to understand my aversion to this technique and how it affected my attitude in the sessions. Since he'd broken his promise, I was always on guard that he would do it again and never felt fully relaxed once he got anywhere near my neck. He did this twice more without warning, but I accepted it because I thought it was the only way I was going to heal.

Sometimes when you ask a question, the universe gives you an answer you may not like. In the moments when the pain seemed so horrific that I didn't know what to do with myself, I would ask *how much worse can this pain get?* Then one day, I got an answer I didn't like. I needed a pedicure and sat on the edge of the tub because I couldn't sit on the floor like I used to since I couldn't use my arms to bear weight and get up, and my legs were too weak. I used to be able to sit on the floor in the lotus position and not use my hands to get up, but now this was physically impossible.

My phone was always close to me because William frequently called from work since he'd had to return after an eight-week hiatus, and if I didn't answer, he freaked out. I was doing my nails when Kathryn texted me. I got up to get my phone, which was on the counter a few feet away, and as I sat back on the edge of the tub, I slipped on a piece of clothing and fell backward and hit my head.

A bit dazed by the fall, I realized what had happened, and when reality set in, the pain at the back of my head almost made me puke. I was flat on my back now, my feet up on the edge of the tub, and I couldn't move. The phone fell into the tub with me, and when I tried to pick it up, it felt like it weighed two hundred pounds. I could barely hold on to it because my hands shook so violently. I managed to call William, and he told me not to move as he was on his way. I thought about the forty-five-minute drive, even longer if there was traffic, and I knew I couldn't stay in that position because my head rested on the bottom of the tub and hurt.

I must have been operating on a double dose of adrenaline because I still don't know how I was able to get myself up. William came home to find me in tears for the pain in my left arm and the big throbbing walnut at the back of my head. As if I didn't have enough to deal with, here I was with additional pain. It was as if the universe was saying, be careful what you ask; you will always get an answer.

I never again asked how much worse my pain could get!

At the end of six treatments with Dr. Aron, three weeks later, I was still in horrible pain. Even though I seemed to feel better during the sessions, the relief didn't last, and I had even worse pain as soon as the same night. On the next treatment, William expressed concern to Dr. Aron that I didn't seem to be making much headway in terms of pain, and the range of motion I'd gotten back in my arms was minuscule.

Dr. Aron said that he would continue the treatments until Halloween, at which time we could decide if we wanted to continue. My spidey senses went on full alert. I knew it was difficult to predict how quickly I should see results, but my instinct was screaming that something wasn't right. I had another three sessions. In my last session, I asked Dr. Aron if he thought I should get new X-rays because I was concerned that I was not healing like I was supposed to. He said it wasn't necessary, and I said okay.

Close to the end of the hour, William came by to get me. As Dr. Aron was finishing up, William asked the same question I had. This time, his response was different, and he said that, yes, we could get X-rays. That bothered me because it wasn't ten minutes earlier, I'd asked the same question and expressed the same concern William had.

I had an uneasy feeling, and it was because I'd broken a promise to myself regarding chiropractors. It's not that I didn't believe chiropractic could help me, especially if the problem were with my spine. But after my first experience with the chiropractor who'd manually adjusted me, I said I would never have another adjustment without first doing X-rays to see what was happening in my body. I let Dr. Aron work with me because we gave him my X-rays from June, but my intuition kept saying that I needed to do X-rays again.

William also agreed that the treatments weren't working as we'd hoped, but more importantly, he felt we needed to do some kind of intervention for pain. I had the prescription for lorazepam and baclofen from St. Michael's hospital, but I didn't want to take antianxiety drugs. As much as I protested, he insisted something had to be done for the pain and filled the prescription. I didn't have much choice in taking it as sleep was now almost nonexistent. He convinced me that it was not something I would have to do long-term, but that I needed rest, even if it was a drug-induced one. He reminded me that the body heals when it rests and that my lack of sleep was making the situation worse.

My first night taking the lorazepam and baclofen was the first night in months that I slept for more than three hours uninterrupted because

I was able to fall off to sleep before the tremors started. I had a love–hate relationship with this drug because, even though I was able to sleep, it made me nauseated the following day. Also, even though I was able to get some sleep, I never dreamed, and that bothered me. I know that, in the whole scheme of things, dreaming didn't seem important, but my life had come to a complete standstill, and dreams were my only way of having any sort of experience. As weird as it might sound, I lived through my beautiful dreams and had exciting experiences when I slept, but now nothing was going on in my life, real or in dreams.

I used to dream of Mom a lot, especially just after she left, and in all my dreams, she was active and having a good time, sometimes even dancing. I would say to her, "Hey, aren't you supposed to be sick?" and she would wink at me or put her finger to her lips and say, "Ssshhhhh!" The sleep induced by lorazepam was a different kind of sleep, and I didn't think I dreamed, or, if I had dreams, I didn't remember them. I took OTC anti-nausea medications to help with the nausea, but it made me so loopy that all I could do all day was prop myself up on the sofa with a cushion behind my back. I could maintain this position for only so long because my neck became sore from holding my head up. The worst part about taking the lorazepam was the ill effects it had on my digestive system.

Not to be uncouth, and it may be too much information, but when I went to the bathroom, I gagged at what came out of me and was bothered by the smell for hours after because it seemed stuck in my nose. My diet didn't change, but I wavered between diarrhea and constipation, and the bloating caused terrible discomfort in my belly. When I started taking lorazepam, I took half, and it worked for a while until it didn't. So, we upped the dosage to one. It again worked for a while, and when I couldn't fall asleep before the tremors started, we again increased the dosage to one and a half. The effect of the drug wore off, and, for the three months I took it, I kept wondering how many times I would have to increase the dosage. I didn't like the path I was on with this drug, and as much as it helped me sleep, I knew I had to get off it.

Getting addicted to this drug frightened me, and the thought that one day I would be so dependent on it that I couldn't do without it concerned me. I'd heard too many stories of people taking prescription drugs for pain or whatever ailment they had and becoming addicted. I didn't want to end up like that. I read up on lorazepam in the middle of the night once, when it didn't work, and the article advised against using the drug for more than four weeks. By that time, I had already taken it for three months. The ironic thing is that my family doctor prescribed a three-month supply after the two-week prescription from St. Michael's ran out. He renewed it again without cautioning me about the potential dangers or that I shouldn't use it for a long time.

On December 31, 2018, I took my last lorazepam and began 2019 with the same old sleep problems, but I was intent on getting this drug out of my system. It was not easy, and I used OTC sleep aids, changing it up, and sometimes used melatonin. I slowly managed to get the sleep problem somewhat under control enough to get a couple of hours of sleep.

ACUPUNCTURE

William cancelled further treatments with Dr. Aron and decided to try acupuncture to see if it would help with my pain. I didn't think it would because, as part of my physiotherapy with Tom, I'd had acupuncture, and it hadn't worked. I couldn't argue with William because I had nothing left in me. We went to the pain-management clinic and met with Dr. Sophia, who'd also had her own experience with a spinal injury, at the same place I had mine, C6/C7. She had fallen down a flight of stairs, and, even though we had some of the same symptoms and pain, she was able to move her arms enough to do acupuncture on herself.

She was enthusiastic about my prognosis and was sure she would be able to help alleviate my pain with acupuncture. She put needles in different parts of my body; legs, stomach, fingers, and navel, and they added another level of pain because of the sensitivity of my skin. The ones that hurt the most, however, were the ones at the base of my skull. The needles didn't stay in, as she inserted and quickly removed them, to relieve the pressure I felt. It felt more like a hot skewer going into my neck.

As usual, there seemed to be some ease, but it never lasted. I wondered if I so wanted it to work that I convinced myself it did until it didn't. The drive to Dr. Sophia's office was over an hour, and getting there was uncomfortable, but on the trip home, all I could do sometimes was lie in the back seat, holding back my tears, so William didn't worry. When we got home, I just collapsed on the sofa from exhaustion and pain.

I didn't know how long I was supposed to do the acupuncture treatments to get any long-lasting relief, but after about six treatments, I said to William that I just couldn't do it anymore. I had been sure things would turn around once we discovered what my issue was, but by the end of October, I was not getting better. There didn't seem to be any hope because I knew Dr. Aron's technique of manipulating tissue and muscle wasn't the answer for me. I was a prisoner in my body and home, unable to go out and do the things I wanted, so the Internet was my distraction.

DETAILS! DETAILS! DETAILS!

One day, as I browsed Groupon on my phone, looking for nothing specific, I saw a deal advertised for X-rays and five chiropractic treatments. The thought *buy it* came very quickly, and it wasn't so much the deal that struck me but that the chiropractor did X-rays and a consultation before working with a patient.

Intuitively I felt (and couldn't get over the nagging thought) that I should have new X-rays. We sort of knew the chiropractor because we met him almost nine years earlier. However, William didn't continue to see him as a patient after the first visit because we found someone closer to home. The chiropractor also knew my family; his cousin was a neighbor of my parents, and I thought that because he 'knew' of me, maybe he would have more of a vested interest in my case. I decided to follow my instinct and buy the Groupon offer because the voice within me kept saying that there was more to know. Within a couple of days, I had an appointment with Dr. Dean for a consultation and X-rays, and I intuitively felt a sense of relief and renewed hope. We were Dr. Dean's last appointment of the day on October 26, 2018.

I didn't have a conversation with him when we went to his office a few years back, but I liked him right away. His energy was contagious, and when we sat to do the consultation with him, I felt his compassion and even anger at the ordeal I had endured for so long. His jaw dropped a few times, and he raised his eyebrows in disbelief at the various incorrect diagnoses. A day earlier, I'd filled out his intake form, which asked questions regarding trauma, like accidents, as well as my medical history.

I told him that I had been in a car accident when I was fourteen when Mom rolled the car one morning as she drove us to school. He laughed when I said that it was a slow roll when Mom made a left at the top of a hill and got an old maternity dress she wore, caught in the steering wheel. She couldn't recover in time, and the car slowly went up onto a huge pile of sand at the side of the road and capsized. It felt like it happened in slow motion, and no one was hurt. We were all able to crawl out of the overturned car and, my brother, sisters, and I even went to school.

The initial consultation lasted almost two hours, and he asked questions about my symptoms. We had brought my X-rays and C-spine MRI and told him I had seen another chiropractor but preferred not to say what his diagnosis was, as we wanted a fresh perspective. He agreed, and by the end of the consultation, I could see the exasperation on his face.

Dr. Dean took full spinal and C-spine X-rays, as well as a new thermography scan like the one I had done earlier in June, but this one was more detailed because I saw the image right away on his monitor. He also measured how I carried my weight on a scale, and even though I was even at sixty pounds on each scale, my shoulders were uneven when he measured how I stood because my pelvis was misaligned. We had to wait another four days to discuss the findings of the new X-rays, and I was so anxious that the four days seemed like four months. I knew there was more to know about my condition, and this would be the turning point in my nightmare. I had a good feeling about our impending meeting.

We were Dr. Dean's last appointment of the day since it would take a while to explain the X-rays and discuss his findings. He had the same diagnosis as Dr. Aron, but this time, the images showed more issues along my spine than we initially thought.

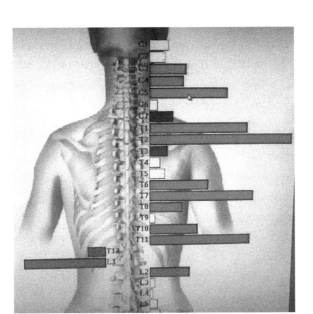

Spinal Thermography (initial visit)

Thermography is a means of measuring the heat (thermos) coming from the body. The science of thermography is the application of these heat readings to locate abnormal pathology or function in the body.[10] I wanted to know more about thermography and learned that,

> The roots of Thermography, or heat differentiation, are ancient, dating back to the time of the pyramids. A papyrus from 1700 BC documents the association of temperature with disease. By 400 BC, physicians commonly employed a primitive form of Thermography: they applied a thin coat of mud to a patient's body, observed the patterns made by the different rates of mud drying, and attributed those patterns to hot and cold temperatures on the surface of the body. Hippocrates summed it up: In whatever part of the body excess of heat or cold is felt, the disease is there to be discovered.[11]

Thermography is used in all kinds of applications to find diseases such as breast cancer, vascular disease, infection, and so on. I learned that

NASA uses thermography as it allows its technicians to see variations in temperature that can be indicative of a weakness or impending failure in a test article. Using an infrared (IR) camera, thermal information is rapidly collected over a wide surface area. The collected information goes through thermal analysis to reveal information such as:

- Electrical and mechanical issues - hotspots indicating loose electrical connections, failing components, improper component installation, overloaded motors or pumps, coupling misalignment, and other undesirable conditions.
- Metal thinning - Material thinning can be observed since heat is conducted away from the surface faster by thicker regions.
- Flaw detection - Flaws can be detected because the flow of heat from the surface of a solid is affected by internal flaws such as disbonds, voids, or inclusions.[12]

My scan shows where interferences are and how much interference is occurring at each level. White shows that signals are getting through to those areas properly like they are supposed to, so the ideal scan shows white all the way through. Other colors represent that signals are not getting through, and different colors represent different amounts of interference. Greens are low amounts of interference; Blues are moderate to medium; Reds are high. There is also a black indicator bar, but he said: "let's not go there." It is important to look at the entire spine because if there is compression on nerves at the top of the spine, signals that come out of that area will be interrupted, and they won't get through to the bottom of the spine, or anywhere else for that matter.

I asked why it showed white at C1/C2/C6 and green at C7 when these areas caused so much grief. The thermography scan doesn't show the damage in the spine, but what is happening at the moment the scan is done, a snapshot that helps pinpoint patterns and whether they are recurring. There are ligaments and tendons on either side of the spine, which help with movement, and when the joints become misaligned, it causes strains that can lead to injuries to the tendons, ligaments, and so on in those areas. When he did my scan, even though signals were getting through at C1/C2/

C6, because I had not moved my neck in months due to the muscle atrophy and pain, it didn't indicate interference with a red bar.

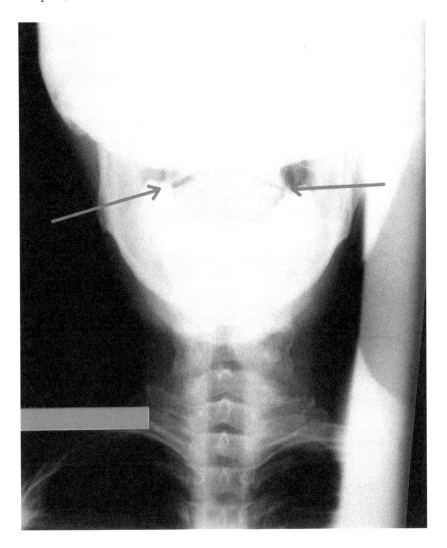

APOM (Anterior to Posterior Open Mouth) X-ray

The actual injury to the spine, however, could be seen on the APOM X-ray. Dr. Dean explained that my C2 vertebra had rotated (along with the C1 because an issue in one vertebra will affect another), and it caused an imbalance in the structure of my spine. These joints were not articulating the way they were supposed to, and it caused the space between C1/C2 to be compacted, and the area is compromised. The two regions indicated by the arrows in the APOM X-ray show the discrepancy in the spaces; the size of the space on the left side (right side when viewed from the front) is potentially compressing my vagus nerve.

He had a model of the spinal cord and showed us the thirty-one pairs of nerves that come out of the spine, and said that each pair connected to a specific region of the body and, ultimately, to different organs.

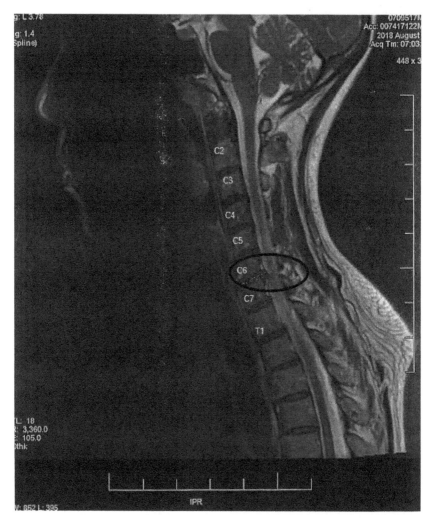

C-spine MRI. C6/C7 was considered unremarkable.

The subluxation (I use the term in the chiropractic sense) at C6/C7 noted on the MRI, was responsible for the pain I felt in my arms, neck, fingers, and the tingling sensation in my hands. He explained which nerve affected which finger, and I understood why the pain in my fingers started at different times. I think my mouth was open the whole time he talked because it was incredible to me how so many doctors had missed it when it all seemed so basic.

I was astounded! All of my symptoms seemed to be related to the problems in my spine. Yet the doctors said nothing was wrong. The combination of my C-spine MRI and X-rays, spinal thermography, and full-body X-rays told the full story of my spine. What wasn't remarkable on one form of imaging showed itself on another. For instance, the spinal thermography didn't show the problem at C6/C7, but the soft-tissue MRI did.

I thought of the radiologist's reports, which identified the issues but saw them as unremarkable and insignificant. My mind raced back to Dr. James, who told William to get me off the medical treadmill. I realized that had William listened to him, I would have eventually lost the use of my legs the same way I had lost the use of my arms. I felt a flush of anger wash over me as I wondered if my family doctor had stuck with me when I first presented with pain in my sides, would we have figured it out sooner.

I had to stop thinking like this and focus more on the road ahead, so I continued to listen to Dr. Dean's explanations. He showed us the X-ray of my full spine and said that it looked like a country road as it veered off to one side. He explained that any deviation of the spine from its optimal position was not good.

I had to ask Dr. Dean the question: "How could the radiologists who interpreted the MRI and X-rays look at something like this and think it was unremarkable and insignificant?" I was astounded that William, with his B.Sc. and two years of medical school, figured it out just by looking at the images, and these doctors (if they looked at them), and radiologists whose job it was, couldn't!

His response was simple, yet profound: "It's Anatomy 101, and they just don't think. We all learned the same thing in school." He said that they look for an actual injury, in terms of an accident, where the spinal cord is severed, and only then is it considered remarkable.

I then said, "But, if a patient doesn't present with issues, and the same thing happens to their spine, then it would be unremarkable. But I had so many symptoms."

He shrugged his shoulders, and I could see that he was just as bothered as I was. I talked about my tremors, and how we'd thought they might be related to menopause but discounted it because of when I got them. We thought the same of the pounding issue because many menopausal women have heart palpitations, but mine was not sporadic; I had it 24/7, and it got worse by something as simple as turning in bed.

We told him we'd learned about the sympathetic and parasympathetic nervous systems and wondered if this could be responsible for my tremors. I wanted to know how these nervous systems worked and how they possibly affected my ability to fall asleep, as well as the constant pounding in my chest and sometimes, simultaneously, other areas in my body.

Even though my symptoms sounded strange and random, I felt I could tell Dr. Dean about them. I said that I had the throbbing sensation in my solar plexus area, head, jaw, cheeks, and teeth. Sometimes it felt like I had mini-hearts all over my body, beating out of sync, and this in itself caused more anxiety, which increased the pounding because I didn't know what was happening to me. My regular resting heart rate was sixty-eight, and it sometimes increased to ninety or higher for no reason, even if I was just sitting watching TV.

I asked him what had caused this to happen to me because I couldn't understand why my spine was so dis-eased. He said it was difficult to tell, and that, most times, there is not necessarily one, but a combination of factors that could contribute to the condition of my spine. He pointed out the accident as a potential causal factor, and I again reminded him that the car rolled slowly, and we tumbled so quietly that no one got hurt. He said one thing he knew for sure was, in his professional opinion, what happened to me had occurred over more than twenty-five years or so. He noted that stress plays a significant role in cervical-spine issues, especially where I had it at C1/C2.

That's when it all started to make sense. I could probably accept that the car accident could have maybe caused the problem at C6/C7, but the other issue at C1/C2, I think, resulted from the long-term, unchecked emotional stress I endured for so long. There is no other possible explanation of why this happened to me.

SUBLUXATION

- A **disconnection** between brain and tissues
- **Robs the body** of health potential by stopping the flow of life caused by stress – physical, chemical and emotional
- It can occur anywhere in the spine but has the most **impact in the upper neck** – the atlas and the axis bones
- It results in **dis-ease and eventually disease**
- It is **corrected** by a specific **chiropractic adjustment**

In Dr. Dean's office, I saw this poster with a more holistic approach, compared to the dictionary definition of the word subluxation, and it clicked. It is common knowledge that stress affects the body, but when I saw this, and specifically how it related to my condition, it seemed to make a whole lot more sense that my most significant issues were in my C-spine, specifically C1/C2, or the atlas and axis. Dr. Dean explained that the spine is like a chain, and when one link (vertebra) is affected, other connecting vertebrae can also be affected. The last eighteen months flashed through my mind, and the next logical question was, "How do we fix this?"

My mind raced back to the reality that we were in a chiropractor's office, talking about spinal issues, and I quickly became aware of the possibility that I would need adjustments. William explained my aversion to manual adjustments, and Dr. Dean casually said, "No problem" and left the room. I looked at William a bit puzzled, and a few seconds later, he returned with a stainless-steel instrument that fit in the palm of his hand.

I exclaimed, "That's it? That little thing is going to fix me?"

He laughed and explained that the results were the same as having a manual adjustment. The adjuster tool precisely targets the area it's used on, and no surrounding tissue is affected *per se* (once the spine moves, so does the surrounding tissue, muscles, and so on.), just the spine.

As he said, tissue, I had an *AHA* moment, as I remembered Dr. Aron's technique of tissue and muscle manipulation to get my spine back to its optimal position. The way I understood it, he was trying to realign my spine (pole) and relieve the pressure on my spinal cord by manipulating tissue and muscles (the ropes). However, it seemed to make more sense to focus on straightening the actual pole (my spine), which would then pull the attached muscles, ligaments, etc. along with it. Dr. Aron's technique may have worked, but I think it would've taken much longer and with a lot more pain. I imagined a carriage with a horse pushing it instead of pulling it. Even though both might eventually get to the intended destination, it would have taken a lot longer and required a lot more effort than if the horse pulled the carriage.

My first adjustment with Dr. Dean was October 29, 2018, and William had to help me onto the adjusting bed. I was a bit nervous because I wasn't sure if this would add to my already aching body; I was way past my threshold for pain, and remembering my treatments with Dr. Aron made me even more anxious. Dr. Dean promised that the adjustment wouldn't hurt, but cautioned that the aftereffects would feel as if I'd worked muscles that I hadn't in a long time.

He used the adjuster tool, at the lowest setting, on different areas on the soles of my feet, calves, hamstrings, buttocks, and along both sides of my entire spine. He was right, it didn't hurt, and it was over very quickly. Every time I was adjusted, I had different reactions. Sometimes I got dizzy right away and had to steady myself when William helped me up, and sometimes I got nauseous. My already lousy headache got worse, and sometimes I felt the pain in my arms as soon as his adjuster tool delivered its burst of energy to my neck. The aftereffects felt different, though. As he said, I did feel like I'd worked muscles I had not in a long while, and I was familiar with that pain. As bad as it was, I knew it was a 'good' pain, so it was more bearable than the other pain I'd endured for so long.

William left work early twice a week to take me to my appointments because I still wasn't able to drive. My treatments took only a few minutes, but our conversations with Dr. Dean lasted much longer as I started my visits with, "So I have a question." Dr. Dean would exclaim, "WHAT!?" pretending to be surprised, then he took the time to explain every question I had. If other patients were waiting or came in during his explanations, he attended to them because my one question usually turned into two or three. I wanted to understand everything I could about my condition and, of course, turned to my friend Google to supplement my knowledge.

Dr. Dean explained that the spinal cord is like a highway. Imagine there is an accident, and three lanes turn into one, or worse, the highway is completely blocked. Information (traffic) slows down and or comes to a complete halt, resulting in a delay in getting to the destination (brain). It works both ways, as the brain sends information via the nerves (highway) to different parts of the body, and it takes information from other parts of the body, back to the brain. Maybe this is why none of the pain meds I took worked, or sometimes even had the opposite effect!

I appreciated the way he explained things, so I understood because I had a hard time processing information due to my sheer lack of sleep and fatigue at this point. He said that the vagus nerve is the longest and most complex of the cranial nerves, and it is sometimes called the wandering nerve. It comes out at the brain stem and is partly responsible for the sympathetic and parasympathetic nervous systems. When I learned more about the vagus nerve, the SNS and PNS, and the effects on these when there is interference along the spine, it made sense that menopause did not cause my tremors.

I wanted to know as much as I could about the vagus nerve and learned that it comes out of the brain and transmits information to and from the surface of the brain to tissues and organs elsewhere in the body.

> The vagus nerve has two bunches of sensory nerve cell bodies, and it connects the brain stem to the body. It allows the brain to monitor and receive information about several of the body's different functions. There are multiple nervous-system functions provided by the vagus nerve and its related parts. The vagus nerve functions contribute to the autonomic nervous system, which consists of the **parasympathetic and sympathetic** parts. Essentially it is part of the circuit that links the neck, heart, lungs, and the abdomen to the brain. The sympathetic side increases alertness, energy, blood pressure, heart rate, and breathing rate. The parasympathetic side, which the vagus nerve is heavily involved in, decreases alertness, blood pressure, and heart rate, and helps with calmness, relaxation, and digestion.[13]

My mind flashed back to the intern at St. Michael's who had done my intake and had looked at me like I had three heads when I told her about my tremors. The clue to what caused my tremors, showed itself specifically in when I got them, and I was clear to anyone who listened that they only happened when I was dozing off to sleep. If they occurred at any other time of the day, it might have been possible they were caused by menopause, like the women William found on the menopause blog.

The burning pain I described down my arms, which stemmed from my neck, also didn't clue in any of the young interns I saw that day, and it took everything in me not to be angry. I chalked it up to them, maybe, not remembering that part of their training, because they supposedly all learned the same thing in school.

Dr. James was an older man, so I assumed he'd been a doctor for quite a long time, and he too discounted my symptoms and didn't make the connection. The fact is that people depend on doctors to know these things, to save their and their loved ones' lives. None of the seven doctors, including the attending one, was even familiar with the kind of tremors I described, whether caused by menopause or compressed nerves, and they sent me on my way with a mental illness diagnosis and antianxiety drugs.

Dr. Dean said the pain in my sides and stomach area, could also be caused by the same vagus nerve, as it has its hands in many areas, and when it is affected, it gets pissed off. Not a very medical description, but I appreciated his euphemism to describe what was happening to me because, as I listened to him, I had difficulty understanding what he said. If he used any of the medical terms I knew he knew, there was no way I would be able to follow him. The first time he used this adjective to describe what nerve interference and its effects could feel like, I agreed because it did feel as if my nerves, ligaments, and muscles were pissed off. The stitch-like pulling pain could also be related to muscle and tissue. When my spine moved and pulled the connecting tissue, muscle, etc. along with it, it would explain why I felt the tightening, twisting sensation. Still, it seemed that all of my symptoms were in one way or another connected to interference in multiple areas of my spine.

He said that the higher up the spine an injury is, the worse the physical symptoms are, and two areas in my C-spine were affected. I also had issues along my thoracic and lumbar spine, which complicated things even more and could also have contributed to the stitch like pain in my sides. The thought of others with the same issues I had, being told by medical doctors that they are making up pain in their heads, made me angry.

Also, when I read the radiologist's report regarding my C-spine MRI, it noted a broad-based osteochondral bar formation.

> An osteochondral bar is a degenerative overgrowth of tissue. When the spine has abnormal pressure of movement of a vertebral segment, the disc, joint, and vertebra will start to degenerate. The disc can either lose height, and water content virtually drying up, or bulge outward from its normal position. The joint/vertebra will start to lay down more bone, which results in spurs and overgrowth that can create these 'bars' of tissue that are comprised of cartilage (chondral) and bone (osteo).[14]

I read somewhere in the many documents I read online that, if an osteochondral bar shows up on X-rays or other imaging, one should seek medical attention, even if there were no symptoms. I wanted to scream *I HAD SYMPTOMS* and kept getting angrier the more I learned. The radiologist noted the issues on my reports, yet discounted them as unremarkable and not significant. My family doctor also received copies of my MRI and X-rays, and he didn't flag any of the issues because he depended on the radiologists' reports.

It seemed like such a waste of resources! I decided to do an experiment as I thought that maybe the doctors and even the young interns didn't remember their basic medical training. I contacted a young lady named Emily, who had just finished medical school barely a month before. She had not yet started her internship, and I thought her medical training would be fresh in her memory because, according to Dr. Dean, they all learn the same thing in school. I sent her a picture of my C-spine MRI and asked if she saw any issues. I didn't tell her about Dr. Dean's diagnosis because I wanted her fresh perspective.

She texted me back and said that she saw an issue at C6/C7, but she didn't think there was anything significant.

Well, there you have it. The newly graduated Dr. Emily made a conclusion based on her recent academic training. She, too, could potentially diagnose someone with a mental illness, if they showed the same symptoms I did. She did say, however, that a radiologist was more qualified to read the MRI. More qualified? *HUH!* I remembered those old medical TV shows where doctors read their patients' X-rays themselves and were able to point out issues of concern. It seems to me that doctors depend solely on radiologists' analyses, instead of looking at the images, which boggles my mind since they learned about this in Anatomy 101. The irony of it all is that it would probably take the same amount of time to open the image on a computer as it does to open and read a radiologist's report. Who knows, maybe it would take less time, as a deduction can be made quickly by looking at an image as opposed to reading a lengthy report.

THE TURNAROUND

B y November ninth, I had a breakthrough! Only four treatments later, I had a twenty-minute stretch where I felt the pain decrease enough that I could quantify the relief. Since the pain in my arms had started, resting or leaning up against anything resulted in excruciating pain, yet there I was, lying down and feeling almost nothing. It was the most delicious thing I think I've ever felt in my life. I didn't know that feeling almost nothing could feel so good.

Even though it only lasted a short time, it gave me hope that this horrible pain would one day be a long-forgotten nightmare. The day I prayed for finally came, and I basked and basked in this zone and used the memory to get me through the next few months of adjustments. I had varying degrees of pain instantly upon getting a treatment and for two days after. I was still in pain, but it felt different.

I had my treatments on Mondays and Thursdays, and I was curious why every time I had an adjustment, I had such terrible pain for the two following days. Then, I would feel better and on the third day, have another treatment, and have worse pain for the next two days. Dr. Dean explained it like this: At my initial visit, my body had been in position A for several years. When I had my first adjustment (and with each subsequent one), my body moves into position B, toward where I am supposed to be. The muscles from position A now had to work slightly differently, as some relaxed while others worked harder. With each treatment, my muscles would generally find a different position which they were not used to, and this was why I felt sore as if I'd exercised (especially after my very first treatment) each time.

It was not always the same, but, generally speaking, I felt pain in different places with varying intensity. I wanted to know how Dr. Dean knew where along my spine to use his adjuster tool. He said that he knew by feeling. "Part of it is by muscle tension, part of it is by joint movement, and part of it you feel by heat or heat differentials." I guess this is the specific kind of chiropractic adjustment I'd read about on the poster in his office.

Regarding the uncomfortable throbbing in my solar plexus area, he said it was most likely because of my compressed vagus nerve since there is a big dissection where the nerve starts to feed the abdominal cavity. I had the same sensation sometimes in the joints of my legs as well. Dr. Dean explained the uneven splits the nerves make, and that I felt it in multiple areas because there are breaks in the river, (my spine), which could cause turbulence along my nerves. He said that, where I felt the sensation of a heartbeat, those are major junction points along different regions of the body, and that's where I could or would feel as if hearts were beating.

About why the beats seemed out of sync, he said that, if I paid attention, it would feel like they went in sequence, or there was a cascade effect as it went along the nerve, and described it as a major contraction. In researching the vagus nerve, I was amazed at the different symptoms one could develop if there are problems with this one nerve because it connects to so many major organs. The following diagram illustrates the number of organs the vagus nerve touches.

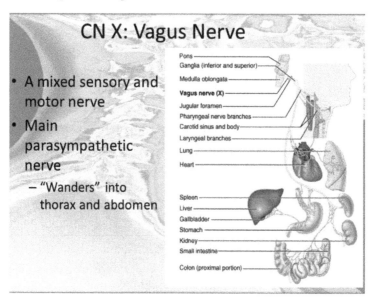

15

I wanted to understand these sensations that had frustrated me to no end and kept me up many nights. Dr. Dean explained that the SNS and PNS run simultaneously, and one becomes more dominant, depending on our environment, emotional state, etc. For instance, if I were sitting watching TV, my PNS would be more dominant, and I would be in a relaxed state. However, if William jumped out from behind the sofa and scared me, my SNS would become more dominant; my heart and pulse rate would increase, and so would the blood supply to my muscles, etc., to deal with the perceived danger.

Things like digestion, for instance, would be put on the back burner because other functions that are necessary to deal with the threat would take precedence. I considered the possibility that, because I've been stuck in the sympathetic state more of the time, as the 'switch' occurred when I dozed off, my nervous system thought there was still danger to deal with, either emotional (psychological stress) or physical (pain). The two systems then 'fought' for dominance, and my body would start to tremor as if to prevent me from going into the parasympathetic state. It was as if it wanted to stay in the sympathetic one because it sensed that it was not safe to rest and tried to alert me to deal with the danger.

I asked if Dr. Dean if he had ever met anyone with the kind of tremors I have. He said that the closest in his experience is someone who gets visible tremors, but they're more like muscle spasms. It's nothing like I have experienced, though. I refuse to believe that I am the only person in the entire world who has these two specific issues and that no doctor has come across them. Even worse, some people potentially have this condition and are being misdiagnosed with a mental illness.

It scared me to even think about what would have happened if I'd continued to take antidepressants to mask my pain, instead of finding and dealing with my actual medical condition. I had minimal movement in my arms, and my legs were beginning to show the same symptoms, and it was progressing very quickly. There's no doubt that I would have become immobilized and dependent on William until my organs failed because my symptoms went unchecked.

If we had listened to those doctors, I would also have spent the rest of my days drugged up on antidepressants and who knows what other kinds of pharmaceuticals, with their hundred and one potential side effects, to mask the pain. At the same time, the root cause of the dis-ease in my body would have slowly killed me. All I could think about was that by the time I passed (or failed) the tests that the neurologist and neuromuscular specialist did, there is no question in my mind that my life would have taken a disastrous turn.

I was sure I was healing, and I knew that it would be a slow process and accepted it. But my thoughts kept going back to the somatoform-disorder diagnosis, and how it could potentially affect the rest of my life. If I ever got seriously ill, let's say with appendicitis and sought medical attention at St. Michael's, when any medical doctor saw my somatoform-disorder diagnosis in their system, would I be taken seriously? When I told a doctor I had stomach pain, they might think it is another made-up symptom of my mental illness.

Kathryn, who has a medical background and loves to do research, told me I should see a physiatrist. It was another term I hadn't heard before. A physiatrist "specializes in a wide variety of treatments for the musculoskeletal system. The muscles, bones, and associated nerves, ligaments, tendons, and other structures - and the musculoskeletal disorders that cause pain and or difficulty with functioning."[16] I agreed it was a good idea because I wanted a medical doctor to see that I wasn't making up pain out of nowhere, but, more importantly, I wanted it documented in my medical records. We didn't get the appointment with the doctor she recommended, but we made an appointment with another physiatrist on her list.

I had a specific reason for going to this specialist, and it was not for a diagnosis, because I was way past that point. I asked Dr. Dean to send a letter to my family doctor for the referral. Because chiropractic services are considered nonregulated primary care, Dr. Dean's diagnosis and treatment doesn't get included in my medical history, which in itself is ludicrous, since it is part of my health history. Why it is that anything relating to my health, no matter if I see a chiropractor or a physiotherapist, isn't included in a central filing system is beyond my common-sense comprehension. (This needs to change!) I didn't know it then, but I came to realize that, generally speaking, many medical doctors do not consider chiropractic doctors or their diagnoses and treatments as legitimate. (More about this later.)

When we went to see my family doctor, it took everything I had in me not to be angry with him. If only he'd listened to me. *Water under the bridge,* I kept saying in my head, over and over. He did the referral as we requested, and we took my X-rays, Dr. Dean's letter, and my C-spine MRI to the appointment. The following is Dr. Dean's letter to my family doctor:

November 12, 2018,

Re: Sherri

To Whom It May Concern:

Sherri   is a 50-year-old woman who presented to the office on Thursday October 25, 2018. Sherri has been facing an overall decline in her health status for approximately the last 19 months that has resulted in, but not limited to, severe pain, reduce active ranges of motion of the cervical spine, and upper extremities. Currently Sherri's health has reached a state where she requires daily help to complete her activities of daily living such as bathing, cooking, and cleaning. As a result, Sherri is unable to hold employment or drive. Sherri is unable to perform the above list daily activities due to the level of pain, with the main area of pain concentrated in her cervical spine and across the tops of her shoulders bilaterally.

Sherri presented to the office with copies of multiple previous X-ray, MRI and CT scan reports. The reports cover the entire previous 19 months with the most recent one having been taken August 27, 2018. Sherri has been to seen several specialists for her declining health, and as a result has several radiology, MRI and CT scans.   Sherri has tried several different changes in medication to find a resolution to her pain with no positive end result, even when trying some very powerful NSAIDS such an OxyContin and Percocet. Medication changes were made due to the ineffectiveness to mitigate the level of pain, or result in any positive motion in overall health.

Upon review of the documentation brought into the office, as well as looking at the set of x-rays that were taken on her initial appointment in the office it can be seen that there are several areas of concern within the nervous system and spinal column.

As noted in the MRI reports there are several areas of the cervical spine where there are degenerative changes, osteophyte formations, foraminal narrowing and central canal stenosis. At some levels the narrowing is noted to be either "unremarkable" or "not significant". Also noted are broad based osteochondral bar formation coupled with further foraminal narrowing. When the individual images of the MRI as viewed it is clear that there are multiple levels of encroachment on the spinal cord in the cervical spine located from the C3/C4, C4/5, C6/C7, and C7/T1 to various degrees.

Lateral cervical spine x-ray shows that there has been a loss of the normal cervical spinal lordosis, resulting in the current state of anterior head posture. Also noted is the reduction in the atlas plane line. There are several areas of degeneration noted in the in the cervical spine especially noted at the C6/C7 level, that is also accompanied with a loss of vertebral disc height, and endplate degenerative changes.

The anterior to posterior open mouth x-ray (APOM) of the cervical spine shows that there is an overall positive alignment of the cervical spine. The issues noted in the APOM x-ray are the left rotation noted of the C2 vertebra, and a noted difference in the size of the spaces within the atlanto-axial joint with a decrease noted on the right side.

The above noted changes through CT, MRI and x-ray all confirm that there is an overall compromise of the spinal cord, the nerve roots and the osseous structures that compromise the cervical spine. Based on anatomy and neurology texts it is well documented that this area of the nervous system is responsible for the control and regulation of the structures, organs and vessels of the face, neck and shoulder region bilaterally. Included in this region of control is the brachial plexus that is directly responsible for the control of the anatomy that is resulting the most pain for Sherri, most notably the control of her upper extremities, resulting in pain, and numbness and tingling throughout the C4 through T1 myotomes and dermatomes. There is no amount of pressure on the nervous system that should be dismissed as "not significant or unremarkable", especially in the cervical spine. Any abnormal pressure, or contact with the nervous system can result in greatly altered function of the muscle, or organs that are associated with the affected region of the nervous system, and to dismiss them as "not significant" is a disservice to any patient.

The resulting compression of the spinal cord cannot be dismissed as a major contributor to the health decline that Sherri is dealing with on a daily basis. The duration of time that she has faced this complicated issue, along with the number of times that she has reached out for help should not be dismissed out of hand. There is a very complicated health issue going on here, and as a team it needs to be addressed in the best, fastest and most efficient manner possible to help Sherri return to her pre-injury activities of daily living. While Sherri at times has not presented as a textbook case for any one stand out issue, that does not mean that her complaints are unfounded, nor should they be dismissed as malingering, or as a quest for more medication. This is a multi-faceted health problem and should be treated, and respected as such.

If you have any questions please reach out to the office for further explanation.

Yours in Health,

D.C.

We met Dr. Shaun at his office on November 27, 2018, at another top hospital, Providence Healthcare. He introduced us to a young man he said was an intern, and I had a déjà vu moment when I remembered the six interns at St. Michael's. I thought, *Great! Another young mind to teach the wrong thing.* Still, I tried to keep an open mind since we hadn't yet started our conversation. The doctor said that he'd read through my test results on his computer and asked how he could help us. We gave him the letter we had from Dr. Dean, and he quickly scanned through it and asked about my experience. He did some of the same tests the neurologist had done and diagnosed me with myofascial pain. He didn't look at any of the imaging we brought, and it was evident very early in our meeting that he was not interested. He'd already gotten his information from my records in the system—the same reports that said my symptoms were unremarkable.

I asked if he believed I had a somatoform disorder, and he disagreed with the diagnosis. That's all I cared about because his diagnosis, if he officially did one, would be recorded in my medical history. Just out of curiosity, I told him about my tremors and asked what he thought might be the cause. He noted in his report that regarding her reports of internal tremors at night, I did note that I am at a loss to explain this symptom. I already knew the answer, but I thought that since his specialty is the musculoskeletal system and associated nerves, maybe it would click, but he didn't clue in at all. I imagined what his reaction would have been if I had told him about the sensation that felt like quivering mini-hearts beating out of sync in my stomach, the back of my head, legs, etc. I didn't tell Dr. Shaun about this sensation because I thought he might change his mind about me not having a somatoform disorder.

William called Christy and requested a copy of Dr. Shaun's report that he sent to my family doctor, and when I read it, the only response I could muster was laughter, but after a few moments, my ears started to burn. I may have watched too many cartoons growing up, and I imagined my face turning red and steam coming out of my ears because I was so mad. He talked about the findings from the tests conducted at St. Michael's, and said, furthermore, there were no specific neurological findings… I did discuss with Sherri and her husband today that of the notes available to me; it appeared that a number of consultations did not show a peripheral nerve disorder. An MRI of the spine showed some mild degenerative changes and no signal change in cord or neural component compression.

Are you kidding me?! I couldn't believe what I read, and he wrote this after reading (or maybe not) Dr. Dean's report that no amount of pressure on the spinal cord is okay. And what about my explanation of my symptoms? They meant nothing to him! Alright, so I did have myofascial pain, but what caused it? He never made the connection or told me what the root cause of my debilitating myofascial pain was.

I'd also asked Dr. Shaun his opinion about pain meds I could use to get me over the hump since I had improvements with Dr. Dean's treatments, but the pain was still intolerable. He outlined guidelines for the nature of my specific pain type, and that these included, low-dose amitriptyline, nortriptyline, and duloxetine, and that this should be trialed over a period of many months. I didn't go back to my family doctor to get any of these medications and decided just to bite the bullet and endure the pain. The idea of putting these drugs into my body, and possibly causing other unwanted side effects, didn't appeal to me. Having to use them for many months while trialed was even less appealing when I thought about how everything I used for pain hadn't worked, possibly because my highway (spinal cord) was clogged.

I was curious, however, and googled his three suggested drugs. They are all listed as antidepressants, but they could be used for pain. Before meeting Dr. Shaun, William spoke to our local pharmacist about my inability to get relief with the pain medications prescribed so far, and she suggested that I may have to use the same drugs he prescribed. She advised that, even though they were antidepressants, they are also used for pain because they sort of 'trick' the brain and its pain receptors.

After I read Dr. Shaun's report and his guidelines for using these drugs, I told William I wanted nothing to do with them. I didn't want to trick my brain about anything; I wanted my body to tell me what was happening to it. I wondered about how many people have spinal issues causing the kinds of pain and neurologic symptoms I have. And how many take antidepressants to mask an actual medical condition, while the root cause continues to go unchecked and get worse over time? All because doctors discount the findings as insignificant and unremarkable. I didn't want to be one of those people, and, as bad as it was, I made up my mind to withstand it, and kept telling myself it would get better one day.

In his report, Dr. Shaun also suggested regular physical activity, as this is recommended to treat my pain and function. I usually walk on my treadmill regularly, and since he didn't advise against any specific kind of activity, I decided on squats to help build my core since I'd gotten some relief from the squeezing in my sides. I did about twenty a day for two days, and on the third morning, I couldn't get out of bed. I had horrible shooting pain in my left lower back, side, left glute, and down my left leg. I needed William's help to get in and out of bed and to sit down or get up from a chair. When he was not home to help, I rolled myself to the edge of the bed and lay on my stomach until I could touch the floor with my feet and push myself up. It took about two weeks to get my normal function again. I told Dr. Dean what had happened when I limped into his office, and he said that I had pissed off my muscles by doing too much too soon.

After seven months of adjustments and a bit of impatience, I asked Dr. Dean if there was a way to quantify, by a measurement in millimeters, the movement of my spine whenever I had an adjustment. I had the image in my head of how my spine had veered off to one side and needed straightening when he'd showed us my full spinal X-ray and described it as a country road.

He said that it wasn't a case of looking at my X-ray and saying it needs to move one centimeter, and if it moves one-tenth of a centimeter with one adjustment, I would need so many adjustments to get it back to its optimal position. He said that, unfortunately, even though there was no way to quantify how much my vertebrae moved, the overall objective was to get my joints moving properly. By allowing the joints to move correctly, it takes pressures off of the spinal cord, and the nerves, which, in turn, would enable my body to communicate more efficiently. Part of the communication process entailed rebuilding, whether it was tissue, ligaments, organs, and so on. Over time, as I got adjusted, it would result in my joints functioning better, and this would allow my body to heal and rebuild itself as the discs would be more able to get the nutrition they needed.

Dr. Dean explained that when there is no longer compression on the spinal cord, it will heal because the signals get better, even though I may not be aware of it. He said that the other important issue to consider is that what I wanted fixed in terms of the things causing me stress (pain, tremors, heart-pounding, etc.) weren't necessarily the things my body wanted to fix first. For instance, my body may know something else is awry, for example, in my small intestine, which had way more priority over pain. This information was comforting and alarming at the same time. After all, I wondered what I didn't know because I wasn't symptomatic yet.

He showed us a cross-section of a single vertebra model with the spinal cord inside and said that when the spine lines up correctly, the spinal cord lies in a canal, not touching anywhere along the inside of the spine. He used the analogy of an extension cord and said to picture a cross-section of it, with multiple cables housed in a large orange plastic coating. Each cable controls something different, for example, temperature, vibration, touch, pain, etc., and everybody's is a little bit different, which is why people present symptoms differently. One person may have pain, while another person may have temperature issues. The encroachment could be in the same area of the spine, but how and where the spinal cord is touched will result in different symptoms.

I remembered Dr. Sophia's injury and understood why she didn't have the same symptoms I did, even though we had an injury in the same area of the spine. He also talked about the nervous system in the general sense and said that we have so many nerves, some of them designed for controlling things, and others for feeling things. Because of this, one can have a country road like I did, but if the part of the spinal cord responsible for feeling is touched, one may never know there is an issue. If the spine touches the part of the spinal cord that controls the function of something (for instance, how well the heart or stomach functions), one may not know something is wrong until it doesn't function well for long enough, and shows the dysfunction with a symptom.

Dr. Dean noted that it is possible that by the time a symptom shows up, the function of an organ could be affected generally in the area of 50 percent, and this is when someone may seek medical attention. I found this alarming because I thought about my stomach MRI, which was deemed unremarkable. By the time any, some, or all of the organs connected to my vagus nerve showed symptoms, they would generally be affected by 50 percent! Again, I gasped at the thought. I researched it a bit more, and all I could say was, "Wow!" The sensory functions of the vagus nerve are divided into two components:

Somatic components. These are sensations felt on the skin or in the muscles.

Visceral components. These are sensations felt in the organs of the body.

Sensory functions of the vagus nerve include: providing somatic sensation information for the skin behind the ear, the external part of the ear canal, and certain parts of the throat supplying visceral sensation information for the larynx, esophagus, lungs, trachea, heart, and most of the digestive tract.[17]

When I read that it provides sensation information for the skin behind the ear, it made sense why I had so much pain when I laid on my side, and my ear came into contact with the pillow. It was reassuring to know that, even though some days I didn't feel like I was getting relief or sometimes felt worse, my body was tending to the most critical issues of which I was not even aware. I knew about the body's innate intelligence and ability to heal itself, but to get to the nitty-gritty details of my specific issue was fascinating. Almost every symptom I had was in one way or another related to the problems along my spine.

At one of my treatments, after a particularly horrid night of tremors, I asked Dr. Dean if he knew of a group of chiropractors who shared information about peculiar symptoms they come across in their practice. Specifically, I wanted to know if another chiropractor ever spoke about the kind of tremors I was having. He said that if there was such a group, he didn't know about it and said something that I found utterly senseless. He said that if he had followed the guidelines prescribed by the association he was involved with, I would have only six treatments with him. I asked why, and he said because their guidelines state that if a patient's issues don't get resolved with six treatments, he had to refer me to a medical doctor.

"WHAT!?" I said. "And who would that be since all the medical doctors I saw misdiagnosed me?"

He just shrugged his shoulders, and we both knew what would have happened if he told me he could no longer treat me after my sixth treatment. (It was then that I realized why Dr. Aron said he would do six treatments, and we could decide what we wanted to do next.) The idea that something that had happened over such a long time would heal in six adjustments was the most outrageous and ridiculous thing I ever heard. The other thing I found disturbing was that, even though I appreciated Dr. Dean for helping me understand my symptoms, he said that chiropractors are not supposed to talk about these things with patients, things like neurology and such. *What an outdated way of thinking?* And the implications for patients like myself, who want to understand what is happening in their body?

For many months after Dr. Dean's and my conversation, I was bothered by the seemingly nonsensical way our medical system works. One day I went to a health-food store to get a couple of items and shared some of my experience with a customer service representative, Gisele. She shared her own experience with spinal issues; hers stemmed from an actual accident. She, too, got the same attitude from her medical doctors, and they discounted the possibility that her problems were spinal and possibly related to her accident. (It was interesting that she had had an actual external injury and she was still not taken seriously).

As we shared our experience with medical doctors and their attitude toward chiropractors, she stated that at a time not so long ago, chiropractors and doctors worked together for the benefit of their patients. In her opinion, this all changed when it seemed that medical doctors became unhappy about the competition chiropractors posed to their practice of medicine. I thought there was no way what this lady said was right and decided to find out for myself. In my research, I realized that Gisele hit the nail smack dab on the head.

I read that In October 1976,

Chester Wilk, D.C., and four other chiropractors (one later dropped out) filed suit against the AMA (American Medical Association). The Wilk suit also named many of the nation's other most prominent medical groups as co-defendants-groups such as the American Hospital Association, the American College of Surgeons, the American College of Physicians, and the Joint Commission on Accreditation of Hospitals. The suit claimed that the defendants had participated for years in an illegal conspiracy to destroy chiropractic. On August 24, 1987, after endless wrangling in the courts, U.S. District Court Judge Susan Getzendanner ruled that the AMA and its officials were guilty, as charged, of attempting to eliminate the chiropractic profession. In 1987 (1), following 11 years of legal action, a federal appellate court judge ruled that the AMA had engaged in a 'lengthy, systematic, successful and unlawful boycott' designed to restrict cooperation between MDs and chiropractors in order to eliminate the profession of chiropractic as a competitor in the United States health care system.[18]

I could hardly believe what I was reading! Also, "The AMA's plan to undermine chiropractic became even more organized with the establishment of the Committee on Quackery in 1963."[19] I gasped when I read, Committee on Quackery! It seems that the fear demonstrated then (and probably even now) by MDs toward chiropractors, was weaponized for financial gain. I also found many websites where chiropractic was discounted and called pseudoscience.

The sad thing is that the very people who doctors swore an oath to help in times of medical crisis are the very ones who will pay the ultimate price, with their health. If the medical profession doesn't incorporate chiropractic care into the mainstream health-care system, patients who possibly have atypical symptoms of spinal issues will continue to be discounted or misdiagnosed. It seems to me that MDs' fears are also irrefutably unfounded because our hospitals are literally overflowing with sick people. They should recognize that there are more than enough sick people to go around. All I know is, my scan and X-rays confirmed my symptoms at exactly the areas where I had problems.

It was comforting, though, to see that this attitude toward chiropractors, (at least in the USA), is changing. It also needs to happen in Canada. I glean from conversations I've had with people about the attitude toward chiropractic care, that things have to change from the top down. Change is already happening at the grassroots level because people now realize how important this mode of healing is. Chiropractors won the war, but the battle continues still, and it might be time that the 'powers that be' put patients first. From my personal experience, even though I was initially afraid of chiropractic adjustments (most people are fearful of the unknown), it is a legitimate form of healing that saved my life, without drugs and the unwanted side effects or invasive surgery.

To pick up where I left off before my brief history lesson, my most uncomfortable and frustrating symptoms were the pounding in my solar plexus, chest, and the tremors. I really can't say what is vibrating in me, the nerve, muscles, or all of it. It's interesting to note that sometimes I feel the vibration in my sacral region. Sometimes this happens as I fall off to sleep, but sometimes I feel it during the day when I am up and about. When it happens, it freaks me out a bit. Undoubtedly, the worst is when I have the tremors up the back of my head because it feels like my entire brain is quivering. The possible reason this happens, in either one or both areas at the same time, is that "the vagus nerve is a craniosacral nerve, meaning it originates in the cranium, but also connects to three spinal nerves in the sacrum (S2-4). The parasympathetic nervous system is referred to as the craniosacral outflow."[20]

I firmly believe that the compression on my vagus nerve causes my tremors and pounding. Even though I'm speculating, it's the only explanation that makes sense, based on when they occur. No doctor, even the specialists, offered any other possible reason (except a mental illness), and none took the time to find out. I found this interesting piece in my research about the vagus nerve:

It is essential in fear management. Remember that 'gut instinct' that tells you when something isn't right? It turns out that the vagus nerve plays a major role in that. The signals from your gut get sent to the brain via the vagus nerve, and the signals from the brain travel back to the gut, forming a feedback loop. What if this loop was interrupted – wondered the researchers in a new Swiss study – would that affect innate anxiety and conditioned fear? It turns out it does. In test animals, the brain was still able to send signals down to the stomach, but the brain couldn't receive signals coming up from the stomach. The research showed that those rats weren't that afraid to begin with (lower level of innate fear), but once they became afraid, they had trouble overcoming this fear even when the danger was no longer present (longer retention of learned fear). This shows that the healthy functioning of the vagus nerve helps us bounce back from stressful situations and overcome fear conditioning.[3]

If the compression on my vagus nerve has been happening for so long, could it be that my loop has been compromised for just as long, and my body has trouble overcoming emotional and psychological fears? I can't say, but it gave me a new understanding of what Philip said: The mind may forget, but the body doesn't.

William saw our family doctor (two years after he diagnosed me with IBS), for an issue that he had, and the doctor asked about me. William gave him an update about my progress but said the tremors didn't seem to be improving. The doctor said that he was at a loss about what caused my tremors, even though William previously suggested the possibility that my SNS and PNS are affected by my spinal issues. I don't know if my doctor tried to find out more about my condition to help me figure out what caused my tremors, but the fact that he didn't say he did, speaks volumes. It would be nice if there is a medical professional who has come across this condition, could confirm our theory about what is causing my tremors and the sometimes erratic pounding in different areas of my body.

On my fifty-first adjustment, I asked Dr. Dean what he thought about combining manual adjustments with the ones I got with his adjuster tool. Sometimes, after I had my treatment, William would have a manual one, and I got so jealous of the instant relief he mostly got. I thought I could withstand it on my back, but not (in no uncertain terms) on my neck. Dr. Dean said that it was a good idea. At my next appointment, he

---

3   See Notes at the end for more information on this study.

incorporated not so much a manual manipulation but more of a stretching exercise that he called sacral distraction.

While positioned face down on the adjusting bed, he put one hand under my hip and the other on my lower-back sacral area, and stretched my back. I instantly felt the pull in my lower abdominal area. It didn't hurt, but the tightening in my legs and stomach area seemed to be more intense for a few days after. As usual, on most nights after I had a treatment, my tremors felt worse, and they also seemed to intensify with this added exercise. He did it for another three treatments, but because the tremors got so much worse, he decided to take a break for a bit and see how things progressed.

He said it seemed as though the added exercise irritated the nerve too much, causing the tremors to worsen. Because my case was so unique, our only option was to play it by ear and figure out the next treatment by how my body reacted to the previous one.

Even before I became symptomatic with pain, things were happening in my body that I was not even aware could be caused by spinal problems, and I never really worried about them. For about two years before the pain presented, whenever I ate too fast or too much (by my standards), my heart would pound and race, and I knew it was time to stop. It still happens, but now I see that the compression on my vagus nerve possibly causes it. I learned about the connection between the vagus nerve and its effects on the PNS, which aids digestion.

Also, even though throughout my life, I'd never had problems napping during the day, suddenly, when I tried to nap during the day, my heart rate increased and woke me. I still can't nap during the day, and I cannot deny that this, too, could be because of my compressed vagus nerve.

The likelihood that my TMJ disorder is related to the problems in my spine also cannot be dismissed. I don't want to get technical, but Dr. Dean said a lot of dentists are now referring their patients with TMJ disorder to a chiropractor because of its potential connection to spinal issues, even if no other symptoms exist.

Concerning the pulling sensation I had on the instep of my left foot, I learned that:

The nerves of the leg and foot arise from spinal nerves connected to the spinal cord in the lower back and pelvis (my pelvis
was misaligned). As these nerves descend toward the thighs,
they form two networks of crossed nerves known as the lumbar
plexus and sacral plexus. The lumbar plexus forms in the lower
back from the merger of spinal nerves L1 through L4 while the
sacral plexus forms in the pelvic region from spinal nerves L4,
L5, and S1 through S4....The medial and lateral plantar nerves
are the two largest nerves in the bottom of the foot. Working
together, the plantar nerves command the many small muscles
of the feet and toes.[21]

Since I also had multiple issues along my thoracic and lumbar spine,
it's undeniable that these interferences are a probable factor in the pain
I had in my left foot, knees, and legs. The connecting muscles, tendons,
fascia, and ligaments, which all have a synergetic relationship with one
another, would also be affected.

Dr. Dean explained that I felt like my arms were locked up because
(apart from the excruciating muscle pain), my tendons, nerves, and fascia
were all sort of stuck. He explained it like this: Imagine there are a bunch
of ropes laid out on your driveway, and it snows, covering the ropes.
If you tried to move them while the snow was still fresh, you would
have no trouble doing so. Imagine, however, that the temperature quickly
dropped, turning the melting snow into ice. How easy would it be to
move the ropes frozen in the ice? That's what happened in my arms and
neck, and the only way to get them moving again was to unlock my
tendons, muscles, fascia, and so on (the ropes) by moving them while
getting my spine back into its ideal position.

About the tingling in my hands and fingers, which was the first
symptom I took notice of, I still don't know how doctors didn't relate this
to nerve interference when testing ruled out diabetes. As for the burning
sensation in my neck and arms, how it didn't alert them (especially the
specialists) that it was, at the very least, possible that my issues were nerve-
related is beyond me; they should have continued their investigations.

Still, Dr. Dean said it is essential to keep in mind that there could be ten people with the same injury at the same places I had, and, of those ten people, some of them or none of them might exhibit similar symptoms, or even other seemingly unrelated ones. My take away from this is how complicated and interconnected the human body is and how important it is for doctors to view patients and symptoms on an individual basis because we are all unique and will exhibit symptoms differently.

One day, I was browsing the MSN website to keep myself abreast of what was happening in the world. I clicked mostly on short articles because I just didn't have the attention span to focus on anything too complicated or lengthy. I saw a slide show that demonstrated different kinds of itches the body experiences and what the probable medical cause of each itch was. Neuropathic itch was the one that piqued my interest because there seemed to be no other explanation for my itchy legs.

I thought maybe it could be an explanation since my spinal nerves were affected by the compression on my spine at different places. The possibility existed that the itchiness could be related to menopause, but the fact that it was only on my legs made me research it a bit more. Everybody knows how annoying an itch is, but what about an itch that, the more it is scratched, the itchier it gets! During the day, I was able to ignore the itch or scratch through my clothes, but at night when I was asleep, I did the most damage to my legs. I scratched so hard that I took the top layer of my skin right off, causing dark pigmentation where I scratched the most.

I delved deeper into more than the short slide show and learned that "neuropathic itching is itchiness triggered by nerves. The itch feels deep, like it's under the skin, making the sufferer scratch, especially hard. With neuropathic itching, nerves in the upper (cervical) spine, likely compressed by vertebrae, cause the itch sensation. What seems like a skin condition is truly a musculoskeletal defect, compressing a nerve to cause relentless deep itchiness."[22]

I sometimes had the itchy sensation on my back, albeit it wasn't as bad as the itch on my legs. The skin on my back developed a sort of weird feeling (which by my standards is not all that weird, Dr. Dean would joke with me), like pins or something rough like sandpaper when my clothes came into contact with my skin. I know I didn't suffer from dry skin because William made sure to lotion me up most nights.

Before I found the article regarding neuropathic itch, I asked Dr. Dean what he knew about it because I wondered if he thought there could be a connection between my itchy legs and spinal issues. When he said that he knew nothing about it, I shared my findings with him at my next appointment. He read what I found and said it was quite possible, and he could see how one could cause the other. I mentioned to him that I'd found it interesting that the article was written not by a chiropractor but by a health writer who was a Ph.D., MPH, and RN.

He responded, "Of course not. If a chiropractor wrote it, nobody would take it seriously!" Not to take away from the writer, Dr. Judi Ebbert, but how sad! Chiropractors, as far as I am concerned, deal with the foundation of our body: the spine. How is it that their knowledge and skill are not considered as necessary by the mainstream medical community? The spine is like Grand Central Station, with nerves bringing messages from and taking messages back to the command center: the brain. The fact that chiropractors specialize in this area of the body is valid and meaningful. Yes, I saw two chiropractors before Dr. Dean, but they both saw my issues and certainly didn't think they were unremarkable and insignificant. Dr. Dean took the time to look at my X-rays, C-spine MRI, and spinal thermography, which told the whole story, and I was able to finally find out what my issue was before it was too late.

On the other hand, I saw **TWENTY-SIX** medical doctors, some of them specialists, and they all (except for the cancer-clinic doctors and the internal medicine specialist) misdiagnosed me over and over again.

As for my sudden weight loss, which had started in late December of 2017, it may be a menopausal symptom. It is also possible that it could be related to the stress of not knowing what was wrong. When I did my stint in Trinidad, my stress levels were so out of control that I lost about the same amount of weight I lost this time around.

On an interesting note, in my research about adrenal fatigue, I learned something even more remarkable about the correlation between menopausal symptoms and the adrenal glands. Dr. Eric Berg talks about the 'mechanism of menopause,' and questions if menopausal symptoms are normal. He says during menopause,

> The ovaries go into retirement, but there is a back-up organ to the ovaries that is supposed to take over because it produces the same hormones as the ovaries. This back-up organ is the adrenal glands. The adrenal glands don't produce the same amount of the hormone, but your body doesn't need that amount of it anymore. The typical menopause symptoms that people say are normal, like hot flashes and night sweats, are not normal. Many women get these symptoms of menopause simply because they're going into it with a weak adrenal (system).[23]

After six months of continued weight loss, it finally tapered off, and I now hover between 120 and 123 pounds. I suppose that, once my stress levels decline (emotional and physical), I will gain some weight. Hopefully! (I chuckled to myself a bit when I learned Dr. Berg is a chiropractor. Even though he has a holistic and quite logical approach to menopause, some medical doctors might be quick to discount him because he is a chiropractor. How insane?!)

Just after we found out what was causing my pain and other symptoms, Kathryn spoke to a neurologist of a friend of hers and gave him a rundown of my symptoms. She said his response was "she's lucky they found out what the problem is because she would have ended up in a wheelchair." I instantly remembered the lady who came into Dr. Adam's office in a wheelchair who had TMJ disorder, and I wondered, *What if she has the same issues as I do!*

In the few seconds it took to digest this statement, my life—if William hadn't kept insisting something was amiss with my spine—flashed before me, and I saw what would've happened. If he hadn't insisted the doctors were wrong, and had we accepted the IBS, fibromyalgia, and mental illness diagnoses, my organs would eventually have been affected. My heart had been beating so abnormally and erratically, who knows what would have happened as time went by. There is no question that my body would ultimately have begun to shut down if I continued to mask my symptoms with antianxiety drugs.

It was only a question of which would come first, failure of my organs, or the effects of sleep deprivation. The first time I heard the terms sympathetic and parasympathetic nervous systems was when Tom used it, and he is a physiotherapist. The second time was with Dr. Tatyana, whose office I never went back to because of her incompetent staff. I question why, if these two professionals got this from a basic description of my symptoms, how was it that specialists, like a physiatrist and a neurologist, didn't know? So, NO, doctor! You are wrong! I don't have IBS (four times)! NO! I don't have a functional disease (whatever the heck that is)! NO! I don't have a somatoform disorder (twice)! NO! I don't have fibromyalgia (twice)! And YES! The results indicated by my X-rays and C-spine MRI are indeed REMARKABLE! FOR ME!

EMOTIONAL JOURNEY

PAIN WILL STEAL YOUR LIFE... IF YOU LET IT!

Pain, relentless chronic pain, be it emotional or physical, will steal your life! If you let it. I know, because it almost stole mine. In 2017, when I first started to have the stitch in my sides, I was still able to live my life because it was more of an annoying discomfort than it was a pain. I described it as a four on a pain scale and a ten on a discomfort scale. For a year, it consistently got worse, and by 2018, it became so debilitating I couldn't perform the smallest of tasks we usually take for granted. Pain changes your perspective on life; it makes you think thoughts you would probably never think under normal circumstances.

I realized the first time I tried weed that I was quickly going down the proverbial rabbit hole when (in crying hysteria), I said to William that I wanted to die. We laid on the bed together with him, hugging me from behind while I cried. The weed was not easing the pain, and I just wanted it to stop. I'd had thoughts of dying before but never let on because I didn't want to worry him, but the weed removed all filters, and I couldn't stop the thoughts in my brain from translating to words from my lips.

I cried and cried, saying to him that I wanted to die. "Please, help me die!" As I turned around to look him in his eyes, to plead with him to please, help me die, I saw that he too was crying. Here was this man who loved me so and made me feel the safest I had ever felt in my whole life just by holding me, and I was the reason he was hurting. It was the first time I ever saw William cry, and this awareness added another dimension of emotional pain. Even though I was high, I became very mindful of the impact my words had on him, and I recognized that he, too, was suffering.

He tried so desperately to help me, and his attempt to ease my pain with weed seemed to make things worse, not because it made the pain worse, but because he saw my true feelings. At that moment, I made a decision that I would never let him see me cry like that again because I couldn't bear to see him in pain. Sometimes I felt like the pain I caused him was worse than my physical pain. I thought I could prevent this kind of pain from happening to him, even though I had no control over how it affected me. I hadn't known men like William existed, and I didn't realize that a man could love a woman the way he loved me. My experience with the men in my life before meeting him taught me things about men that I thought were normal, like dishonesty and physical and emotional abuse.

In my first relationship in my early twenties, I'd experienced a kind of verbal abuse that made me shut down while it happened; part of me knew that someday it would've escalated to more than that. I stayed in the relationship for over four years, even when only a few months after meeting, my first boyfriend at the time cussed at me in public because I didn't do what he told me to. People watched as he shouted profanities at me, saying that I didn't listen to him. I saw the pity in their faces while I shrugged my shoulders and pretended that he was some madman I didn't know.

He got so angry at times that he punched holes in the wall, and my brain just shut down, incapable of saying anything as my body trembled with fear of what he would do if I could even muster a response. One time, as he argued about something, I sat quietly and listened to his rant. When I didn't respond, he came over and held me by my shoulders and violently shook and yelled at me to say something. All I could say was, "You are yelling. What am I supposed to say?" as calmly as I could, and this made him even angrier. I wasn't deliberately trying to anger him, but my brain just stopped working. I think part of me knew that it was safer to keep quiet. I had a lifetime of knowledge of what the consequences would be if I were to respond in any manner or defend myself.

I knew I couldn't have a conversation with someone who was that angry, and I knew it would have made the situation worse. I tried to end it a few times but was always reeled back in with apologies and his promises to change. One time, I made up my mind to get out of the relationship because I knew it was unhealthy, and he cut himself on his chest. When he told me what he had done, I went back for fear that he would hurt himself more. When I went to look for him, after I was unable to get in touch with him for a couple of days, I walked around his neighborhood and found him sleeping on a bench, without shoes. He convinced me that he couldn't live without me and that he would change, so I continued in the relationship, knowing deep down that I was in danger. I grew up seeing violence and knew all the telltale signs, yet I was helpless to get out of the relationship.

I didn't tell Mom or anyone about my experience because I was embarrassed and, I loved him and wanted to protect and help him work on his anger issues. It was during this relationship that I started to sort of understand why Mom stayed in her marriage, even though she was not happy. It finally ended when he asked me to move in with him, and I said no. I saw myself reliving Mom's life, stuck in an abusive relationship, and it scared me to no end. I knew that, once we lived together, it would be that much harder to leave, remembering my mother's multiple attempts and failures to do so. I didn't know how to be strong enough to end the relationship despite my gut instinct, which screamed, get out before it's too late!

And what about children? How could I bring children into a relationship like this? If he could cause physical harm to himself to manipulate me, then what would he possibly do to children?! The idea of bringing children into the relationship and having them be part of the same kind of violence that had such an impact on my life, and experiencing the things I did as a child, was terrifying. I knew (like Mom) I wouldn't be able to protect them. I had to end the cycle! I made decisions out of fear, and, when I look back, instead of feeling bad, I remember what Mom told me. She would say, "Never look back and have no regrets because you did the best you could with what you had."

Not long after I told him that I wouldn't move in with him and his male roommate, he left the country and went back to France (where he was originally from) without telling me. I found out when I called his home one day, and his roommate said that he'd left the country. I never saw him again and am thankful I didn't have to potentially experience the leaving and going back cycle that I had seen for most of my life.

My second relationship was with a man who cheated on me, and I found out when his girlfriend found my phone number in his phone book and called me to find out who I was. When I sought support from my brother at the time, his response to me was, "All men are dogs." It was quite ironic he said this because dogs are very loyal, and I felt his viewpoint gave dogs a bad name.

I knew at the time, however, that his attempt to comfort me was more about his actions rather than men in general, and I focused instead on the advice of my mother: "Not all men are the same. There are good men out there." Mom knew the role models I'd had growing up, starting with my father, so she tried to teach me that, despite her experience and others I saw growing up, there were indeed good men who would treat me with respect.

Even though I didn't tell her about my experiences in my relationships, somehow, she knew they were not right for me, and she let me know. I asked why she felt that way, and she said she just knew. Who wants to admit to their mother that she was right about their chosen partner? So, I kept my secret from her. I need only two fingers to count the number of positive male role models I'd had growing up, where I saw a man respect a woman who was not only his wife and life partner, but also his equal and treated her as such. However, I thought this kind of relationship was the exception rather than the rule. However, Mom always reminded me about the good men out there. As much as I didn't take her advice and end either relationship when she expressed her concerns to me, I secretly took her warnings to heart. Looking back, I wonder if, having witnessed disrespect more than respect in the relationships I observed while growing up, did I attract the same because it was all I knew?

I was forty-two years old when I took Mom's words to heart and started to believe there were good men out there. I remembered that she said her mother warned her about her choice with my biological father because she was so young and he was much older, but she didn't listen. I always had this information at the back of my mind, and even though I didn't at the time, I knew that, at some point, I would have taken her advice. At some level, I knew she was right because she had developed an understanding through her life experience. She didn't have the life experience to guide her choices when she was young, but her mother did and gave her two cents' worth of advice. She was right, according to Mom. From my experiences so far, I knew I had to break the cycle!

Before I met William, I was in a waiting room somewhere, and I saw, if I remember correctly, Oprah's 'O' magazine on the coffee table. I picked it up because there's always something to learn with Oprah. As I thumbed through it, I saw an article about how to attract the kind of partner you want. It said to write one hundred traits you want in a life partner. I thought to myself, *ONE HUNDRED? Who can come up with a hundred things about someone!?*

I laughed it off, but after a few days of thinking about the article, I decided to do it as an experiment. I was surprised when I started to write the list and was able to come up with a hundred things I wanted in a partner. Maybe it was a coincidence that it all happened the way it did, but I think this exercise changed a lifetime of false beliefs I had about men. I also think, at a subconscious level, I internalized and believed what Mom said to me growing up, despite my experiences with the men in my life.

As I wrote my list, I think something shifted in me, and I started to believe that, just maybe, I could somehow find one of these good men with the traits I listed. I wrote my list in a little notebook, tucked it away in my purse, and pretty much forgot about it. Within a couple of months of doing the exercise, William and I met. What makes it even more interesting is that the article suggested being very detailed, for example, what the person should look like and so on. I had a celebrity crush at the time, and even though I did it as a joke, it was a test to see if 'the universe' would deliver the person with the exact traits I wrote down—if the person showed up at all.

The first trait I wrote was spiritual a must, and the second was the name of my celebrity crush, whom I thought was handsome. I wrote both his real name and his screen name, with the words look-alike and a little smiley face in brackets next to it. It so happens that William has the same name as my crush's screen name. Could it be more look-alike than that? It was as if I'd gotten a sign, saying, this is what you requested! Here you go! Coincidence? M-a-y-b-e. I still have the list and use it as a reminder of the power of thoughts and words. The first time Mom met William was at my parents' home. After our visit, as we drove away and waved goodbye, she stood in the doorway and gave me two thumbs up. I knew she was okay with him.

William was different. I knew it from our first conversation, and he has proved it to me in the ten years we've been together so far, and I didn't want to be the reason for his tears. I didn't have to tell him I was in pain because he knew I was. But as far as I was concerned, he didn't need to know the varying levels or the intensity. Like a typical man, he wanted to fix me, but because we didn't know what we were dealing with before my diagnosis, he couldn't, and I knew he felt helpless.

We slept in separate beds because we couldn't risk him turning in the middle of the night and inadvertently dropping his arm on me, which he had done quite frequently before, or even hugging me in his sleep, forgetting my condition. My favorite time of the day had been when we went to bed, and as I turned onto my side, he would hug me from behind and kiss me exactly five times on my back and say, "I love you." Then we would both fall asleep. His breath on my back was soothing, and, as I dozed off to sleep, I marveled at my luck in sharing my life with this amazing man.

Things change, though, and I appreciate that. But when one becomes used to something, so life assuring and comforting, it's hard to get used to anything else. He would tuck me in at night in my separate bed he had warmed up with a heating pad to help soothe my aching arms, neck, and back. It took everything for me not to let him see the tears as they welled up in my eyes, knowing that in a few seconds, I would be alone.

For months, he helped me get into bed, kiss me three times and say, "I love you, I love you, I love you, to the moon and back, infinity and beyond, forever and ever, amen." He held my hands and told me not to give up because, "If it is the last thing I ever do, I will find out what is wrong with you." Every time he walked away from me, I felt like something died inside me because I felt so empty and alone when he went to the other room. I knew he felt the same way, but I was too wrapped up in my pain to think about it then. Besides, I would be awake for much longer than he would, and I would feel the emotional sting for a longer time.

Yes, I knew that rationally speaking, we couldn't be together in the same bed, but the kind of pain I was in made my loneliness feel worse. All I wanted was to be in his arms and fall asleep together like old times. That pain I felt was visceral, and it seemed so much worse than the physical pain and so deep inside, a place I couldn't reach, and the tears just flowed and flowed.

I thought my death wouldn't only be the end of my pain, but it would solve William's as well. I didn't want to go on being the reason he was hurting. I walked in his shoes, and I could only have imagined the fear he felt, not knowing what was wrong with me. If I thought that I could die from this thing that had no name, I knew he was afraid of the same thing, even though he believed he would figure it out. I knew he too felt the sting of lonliness because he couldn't wrap his arms around and comfort me. I loved him too much to be the cause of his pain, and I was willing to give him up, so he didn't have to continue watching me in agony. I knew his life would change, and he would miss me, but he was the strongest man I knew, and I was sure he would be okay.

I confirmed that I made the right decision about hiding my pain when William told me of a conversation he'd had with someone about his experience watching his wife in pain when she was ill. Her husband said that watching his wife suffer in agony was so distressing that there were times he felt like he wanted to end his life, and the only thing that stopped him was that they had children. When we saw Dr. Sophia for my acupuncture treatments, she also shared her experience with pain and how she'd dealt with it. She said that she didn't want her husband to see her cry, so she went to the basement and secretly wept there.

I didn't think I could ever again feel such a deep yearning for something, but pain will steal your life *if* you let it. On those nights, through the relentless crying, I begged God to please let me die. I said I had felt the love of a mother, forgave my father and brother, and helped a few people along the way. I said I had awe and appreciation for my world and my body, but I'd had enough and wanted out. I thought I understood what true love is, and I gave thanks for the wonderful man in my life, but I couldn't go on feeling so lonely in bed by myself.

Months went by, and every day I found myself alive and in pain. Admittedly, I thought, God knew how much pain I was in, so I didn't have to explain anything. I was so scared about my future, and it was terrifying to think about what my life had become, and would continue to be. I then negotiated with God, that if I had to live, to at least take away my pain. I just wanted it to end! There was only one other time in my life I ever asked, begged, and beseeched a higher power for something so fervently, and that was the night I prayed in front of that newspaper clipping when I was seven.

When my prayers went unanswered, in desperation, I called on my dead mother. I told her that if she truly loved me, she would help me die because I couldn't live this way. I said I wasn't afraid of death, as it would be a welcome reprieve; that I was more fearful of living the rest of my days, not knowing what was causing my pain. Feeling alone in bed was more than I could bear because I couldn't sleep with the love of my life and feel his reassuring arms around me.

I didn't consider the fact that Mom couldn't help me die, but pain makes us think and do things we wouldn't usually think or do. As the months went on and the pain got worse, and my cries went unanswered, my desperation turned to anger. I became angry at Mom and God because I felt there was no way either of them loved me as I thought they did. If they did, how could they ignore my pleas for help?

I put the pillow over my head to stifle my cries because I didn't want William to hear me. He would have to work the next day and needed his sleep. I cried for hours until there were no tears left, or until I got to the brink of exhaustion and dozed off; that is if I was able to get past the pounding and tremors, only to be awakened not long after with either the pounding or pain somewhere in my body.

One morning, when I woke up alive (yes, I deliberately wrote this, because it's how I felt when I opened my eyes), I realized I was not going to die—well, not as soon as I was asking to anyway—and decided I would be more proactive. There are different perceptions about suicide, and I had my own beliefs shaped by an innate understanding, which made me contemplate the option. I feel compassion for people who commit suicide because no one but them knows their pain. I didn't have to imagine the trauma of a kind of pain so horrible it makes one think the only way to get relief is by ending it all.

I lived with not only the physical pain but the emotional anguish as well, and it was a close finish as to which one was worse. Having this experience for so long, without an end in sight, made me feel like I didn't have much of an option if I were going to get some kind of relief. Pain meds didn't work. I couldn't seek any other medical interventions, and the thought of living this way for even another day was too much to bear.

I researched the least painful way to end one's life because I didn't want to add more physical pain to what I already had. I had access to a lot of drugs because of prescriptions we filled but didn't use. I researched how much of a particular medication I would have to take to die quickly, with the least amount of pain.

One night when I couldn't take any more, I went to the medicine cabinet and found my lorazepam bottle was not closed tightly, which William usually made sure of because I couldn't open it on my own. I emptied the entire bottle of pills into my hand and stared at them for what seemed like a very long time. I imagined what my body would do if I took them and imagined how sweet death would be because I wouldn't feel any more pain.

I was familiar with stories of people accidentally dying from carbon monoxide poisoning as the car ran in the garage. I researched the kind of death this would bring, and if it would be painful. When I was still able to drive, I would regularly use side roads where there were ongoing home construction projects. Sometimes when I saw a Mack truck in the distance in the oncoming lane, I fought with myself not to speed up and turn the steering wheel a few inches to the left and hit the truck head-on when I imagined how quickly it could be over.

On one of the nights when the tremors made the back of my head and brain feel as though they were quivering, out of sheer frustration, I hit my head in the temple repeatedly, hoping I would die from the blows. When it didn't work, it just added to the frustration I already felt. If it is possible to commit suicide this way, I don't think I had enough strength in my arms and hands to hit hard enough, but the blows were sufficient to cause my throbbing head to hurt even more.

Because I believe we have the ultimate choice over our existence, contemplating ending my pain by taking my life seemed like a viable alternative to living the way I was. I also didn't think death would be the end of me if I chose to ultimately end one life, because I know my soul is eternal.

On one of the many days when I had nothing but time to consider my options, I remembered my perspective on the soul's journey, gathered from various books I'd read over the years. I learned and believe that my soul is on a journey of self-discovery and growth throughout multiple lifetimes. What I don't figure out in one lifetime, I believe I will figure out in another. I don't have any empirical evidence to prove this, but I had to believe in something.

It then dawned on me that, if there was a chance that this is true, I had to conquer the thing causing me so much physical and emotional grief in this lifetime. I thought if I didn't, I was sure my soul would ultimately want to have similar experiences in another lifetime, to learn the things IT wanted to learn by having these experiences in the first place. I don't expect anyone to agree with me; it was just part of the thought process that prevented me from going through with ending my life.

I changed my thoughts from dying to living because I had this vision of my soul, analyzing my life after I'd ended it. The idea of IT not being happy with my decision and deciding to give it another go, with similar kinds of experiences in another lifetime, I will admit scared me and gave me a serious wake-up call! Fear of something is not necessarily a bad thing, and I made up my mind to live. I felt that if my soul wanted to learn specific lessons, and my experiences so far allowed me to learn these lessons, I didn't want to go through comparable experiences again. I was sure there were many other things to learn, but I made peace with the pain and embraced everything I chose to learn about in this lifetime.

I thought about people who chose to end their earthly experience, and I could never judge them because I felt that anyone who ultimately decided not to continue on their journey in any given lifetime, had an inner strength of which they were unaware. When I remembered my view about how strong I believed these individuals were, I thought I must also have the same inner strength.

I told myself that, if I held on for just a little longer, admittedly I didn't know how much longer, and directed the courage and strength I was going to use to end it to get through it, I would come out the other end okay. It was not the easiest thing to convince myself of, but the more I thought about it, the more it made sense. That I chose life in my darkest moments of contemplating suicide was a conscious choice, albeit not an easy one.

Choosing to live physically was not enough, however, and I realized I also had to change my thoughts. As much as I decided not to do the physical act of committing suicide, I knew that if I continued with the negative thinking, I would have accomplished my goal of death, but it wouldn't happen as fast as I wanted.

Part of me knew I was going to die, not necessarily from what caused my pain but from the negative thoughts about giving up. I remembered my thoughts had power to them, and according to Bruce Lipton, "a new understanding of the universe's mechanics shows us how the physical body can be affected by the immaterial mind. Thoughts, the mind's energy directly influences how the physical brain controls the body's physiology."[24]

I thought if my body was listening to my thoughts (after all, everything is energy) and it heard I wanted to die, I was sure it would yield to my pleading. Possibly, other medical issues might have developed because my body would have to start the process of breaking down to grant my request to die. However, because everything takes time, I knew that it was going to take much longer and with a lot more suffering than I could bear.

After learning about the effects of compression on my vagus nerve and its connection to so many organs, I probably would have died a premature death. Still, I would have suffered incredibly before that happened. I had to do something different! The only control I had was over my thoughts, and it became a second-by-second, minute-by-minute, hour-by-hour, and day-by-day exercise to stop the negative thinking.

Another reason I didn't go through with ending my life was, the thought of William coming home to find me dead was heart-wrenching. One night at the dinner table, he expressed that many times on his drive home from work, he expected to find me dead. When I'd stood by the car in the garage, with one hand on the door handle, and the keys in the other, thinking about the sweet relief of dying, I envisioned William's reaction when he returned home from work, opened the garage, and found the car running with my dead body inside. I couldn't do it! I couldn't bring that kind of pain to someone who loved me so much and who I also loved.

I felt so trapped between not bringing pain to William and ending my own, and a constant battle churned within me. When I researched suicide on the Internet, I didn't have the common sense to delete my search history, and William told me he had seen my searches about suicide. I couldn't even imagine what he felt! I walked in his shoes for a moment and felt horrible, knowing I was the reason for his fear day after day. How could he function at work? Thinking about the possibility of finding me dead when he got home must have caused him indescribable anxiety. I remembered the times I'd driven to visit Mom, when fear gripped my body and how awful I felt.

He said that, sometimes, he half expected to find me dead in bed in the morning after overdosing on pills during the night while he was asleep. Before he said this, one day, the pain was so unbearable that I dragged a chair and climbed up to find my lorazepam. The bottle, this time, was closed tightly, and I couldn't open it. I looked to the top shelf of the cupboard to get the bottles of pills he put high, probably thinking

I couldn't reach them, and as I picked up each bottle, I realized they were all empty. He had gotten rid of what we didn't need.

If I wanted to, I suppose I could have smashed the bottle open when he was at work, but the thought of him finding my dead body and living with that memory for the rest of his life bothered me. I told myself that I couldn't have him clean up my mess. Even though I relished the idea of not feeling my pain, I had to make my love for William bigger than my need to end my misery. If he believed he would find out what my issue was, how could I dash those hopes by ending my life?

I am so sorry I put William through that kind of fear, and it's the one regret I do have. When I learned how he felt, I knew I had to change my attitude, but it was not the easiest thing to do. He stayed home with me for over eight weeks, but he couldn't watch me 24/7.

I think the only difference between people who choose to end their life experience and those like Mom, who 'check out,' and me, is that I had the audacity to hold on for a little while longer. I didn't know how much longer or how things would turn around, but I decided to hold on. As a young child and later as an adult, I laughed when my mother often told me that I was stubborn and said that I had to "burn to learn." She'd try to give me advice about something, and when I did the opposite, she reminded me about my stubbornness. I know, however, she would agree with me that this personality trait has served me well in this instance.

As much as parents and friends try to give us the benefit of their experience and an objective vantage point, I believe we don't heed their warnings because it is our innate wish to experience the things we do—for our growth. So, if it were not for my stubbornness, it would have been more challenging to change my thoughts from ending my life to choosing life. Long after I decided to direct my thoughts elsewhere, I remembered Schwartz's view about suicide. He wrote that to lose a loved one is always painful, but

> *When that loss comes as the result of suicide, the pain sears to the very core of one's being in a uniquely excruciating way. Nothing is ever again the same. Often, the people left behind are wracked by guilt and self-blame, and they may feel anger toward those who ended their lives.*[25]

My thoughts shifted beyond the image of William, finding me dead to him having to tell Kathryn that I'd ended my life. She knew more than anybody the severity of my issues, and the thought of him having to make that call to tell her I had ended my life was horrifying. Then the responsibility of her having to explain to the rest of my family troubled me. Even though I didn't have a relationship with my father and brother, I was sure they too would be hurt by my decision. What about my friends who loved me? If I had a phone conversation with someone, I wouldn't talk about my situation, and I mostly stayed away from family gatherings. Since we didn't have a diagnosis, I didn't want to have conversations with anyone about my dis-ease every time I spoke to them. Experiencing it was bad enough. I didn't want to talk about it as it would have taken more energy than I had to expend.

Then there were the what-ifs. What if my attempt at ending it all didn't work? What if the carbon monoxide didn't kill me but damaged my brain, and I couldn't function? What if the pills didn't work, and I ruined my internal organs, or worse, something detrimental happened to my brain?! What if I hit the truck head-on, didn't die and sustained injuries that left me paralyzed? And what about the poor truck driver who would be traumatized for life? I remembered conversations I had with William about the psychological trauma faced by locomotive engineers when people committed suicide by jumping in front of an oncoming train. They were so distressed by what they saw they could no longer work. One time, I even considered using my bathrobe tie to hang from the railing. What if I broke my neck, didn't die, and lost all use of my arms and legs? The way my condition was progressing, it seemed that this would soon happen, but I told myself, at least, for the time being, I was still able to walk and talk.

I already felt like a burden, what if I became 100 percent dependent on William? I had a hard time depending on him as much as I did because I wasn't able to shower or dress myself or prepare my meals. I couldn't deliberately put him in a situation like this! I am glad I had the what-ifs; because I understood the varying degrees of possible outcomes, I wasn't willing to play the odds. Almost daily, it felt like my circumstances tested my faith, and some days it didn't feel like I would pass. I used to read and listen to inspirational stories, but because of my lack of sleep, my attention span was severely limited; I couldn't concentrate on anything for more than five minutes, and when I tried, it just made me more anxious.

My anger toward Mom for what felt like abandonment didn't help. I missed her more than I ever had, and I fought off the longing to feel her holding and comforting me the way only a mother could. I deliberately forced myself not to think about her and purposely blocked any memory that tried to squeeze itself into my mind.

I had to do something different and decided instead, to let Mom in by remembering the experience I had after she transitioned, when she held my face in her hands, and we danced and laughed in mid-air. I focused more on the many times we were in her bed together, when I held her hands, knowing that the reason I did this was so I could draw on the memory of her when she left this world.

IT'S ONLY FOR A MOMENT!

don't have a list of things I did to get through the excruciating physical pain and the resulting emotional turmoil I experienced. I didn't know how to deal with the emotional blowback of feeling discouraged and lonely. My wish for anyone who has attracted this book into their experience and is having a hard time dealing with pain, whether it's physical or emotional, is that you have at least one loved one in your life and can gain strength from their love. William encouraged me every day when I wanted to give up and kept reminding me that we would figure out and fix the issue.

In the moments of terrible pain, I knew that seeing me in pain and unable to help took a toll on him, and I didn't think to ask him how he was. Even though I knew that, if I did ask, he would've said not to worry about him and that he was fine, I'm sure if I'd asked, he would have appreciated that, even in my situation, I still thought about him. I was so wrapped up and so overwhelmed with hopelessness that I didn't ask how he was. There were times I felt like such a burden and apologized when I needed his help to do the smallest of tasks, like putting my hair up. He kept reminding me that he loved me; I was not a burden, and I had to stop using that word. I still felt like it, but after a stern warning one day, I stopped saying it and, instead, felt gratitude for every little thing he did to make me comfortable. Focusing on what I had, the love of another human being, made it a little easier to endure.

As much as William loved me and is my best friend, I couldn't share my deepest feelings of despair with him because I knew he worried about me. He provided for every physical need with love and dedication and, for months, did all the household chores: grocery shopping, cooking, laundry, all the things I couldn't do anymore. He made us dinner every night after working at a stressful job, while all I could do was sit and try to hold back tears for the pain and my inability to help.

Once, at breakfast, he saw how difficult it was just lifting the cup of tea to my lips and brought me a straw, so I didn't have to endure the pain. He knew how much I loved my one cup of tea in the morning, and to have it tainted with pain took away one of the very few things left that I enjoyed. He cut up my food if I needed it, and he talked to me through dinner about being strong and staying positive. His commitment to me was nothing short of amazing, as he helped me to shower and wash my hair because I couldn't lift my arms. When I couldn't stand the heat of the hairdryer on my already burning neck, he laid me on the bed with my hair hanging off the side and dried it that way.

He helped to get me dressed when I couldn't pull my pants up or put a shirt on by myself. The days when I could withstand the pain, he drew me a lavender bubble bath with Epsom salts, lit candles, and played soft music when I got home from my treatments. He helped me in and out of the tub, dried me off, and put me to bed when I could barely hold myself up from the pain and the effects of the warm Epsom salt soak. He never stopped fussing over me, and his dedication to providing for all my needs consistently for months proved that he was all in till the end.

I watched him most Sunday nights as he slumped onto the sofa around eight or nine, exhausted from working a full-time job during the week, taking care of me, and getting chores done on the weekend. When I started treatments, he always made it home early, to take me first to Dr. Aron and then to Dr. Dean. He attended to the smallest of my needs, like pulling up the zippers on my winter boots or putting on my seatbelt because I had no strength or range of motion in my arms to complete these small tasks.

Hiding my pain from William, however, became a full-time job, as I cried all day, hoping to get all the tears out before he got home from work. When he let me know he was on his way, I washed my face, gathered myself, and took the time it took him to get home to get presentable. There were days I cried so much that the back of my head felt as if it would split open. At times, I had to choke back the tears because using the muscles required for crying caused my headaches to worsen. Some days, the tears ran down my cheeks, and I wasn't even aware it was happening.

As much as I tried to hide my tears and be positive and upbeat, some nights at the dinner table, I couldn't hold back, and the tears just flowed and fell into my meal. The visible tears were terrible enough, but the silent, hidden ones were the ones that stole my strength. At least when the tears come out, there is a sort of release, but when they remained inside, it felt as if it added to the pain already eating away at me.

I had a difficult time dealing with my 'poor me moments.' Oh, I had those moments, and it was a daily, moment by moment struggle not to have them. I was very mindful of how different my pain felt when I wasn't feeling sorry for myself. My physical pain didn't ease, but my ability to endure it seemed to diminish. There were times I felt like I was on the verge of going down the rabbit hole and used Bach's Rescue Remedy to help with the depression and anxiety. William made sure I took it every day, and, as much as it helped, the kind of hopelessness I felt, not knowing what was wrong, could be tapered only so much, and the feeling was always just below the surface. William was as supportive and compassionate as he could be, but in the end, the thoughts were in my head, and only I could control them.

Of course, William was empathetic, and yes, we had conversations about my pain, but it was always positive, saying things such as, "You have to get better because the best is yet to come!" Or "You have to get better because we got too much sh!t to do!" I'm not saying this realization meant that everything was all roses because, even as I write this book, I struggle with my thoughts when the pain gets to me.

One day I chatted with my friend Sandy, who talked me off the ledge as I sat in the car having a meltdown in the mall parking lot. When she asked how I was, I responded, "Some days good, some days better." I was very conscious of how my attitude on any given day, either made it a good day or a better day. I told her that I believed I would get better, and she asked, "How do you know you will get better?" I said I didn't know, but my BELIEF that I would, in itself, made a difference in how I felt.

Because not many knew about my condition, I went into hibernation and kept to myself. One of my most loyal friends Donna, who I've known for years, called me regularly on the days it seemed I needed it most. I felt her concern with every phone call because she didn't have the technology to call for free. Still, she called me regularly to see how I was. There were days I needed to distract myself with someone I could be open with, and she always seemed to call just at that moment. It was uncanny, but I understood why it happened.

I watched a documentary once where scientists wanted to know how thoughts connect people. Two individuals were ten thousand miles away from each other, and each had heart and brain monitors installed onto their bodies. When they thought about each other, they both had practically the same heart rhythm and brain waves. I am sure you've had an experience when you thought of someone, and right at that moment or not too long after, your phone rang, and it was that person. What this shows is how interconnected we all are and the power of our thoughts.

There were days Donna prayed with me on the phone, and, through my tears, I told her I was mad at God because I felt so abandoned. She would say, "It's okay, be mad, God can take it," and without skipping a beat, continued to pray. Once, I told her there was no way there is a God because how could God let one body have so much pain, especially when I was asking so desperately for help. After all, we are supposed to ask and receive. She reminded me that my not believing in God's existence or assistance didn't affect God's presence or support and that God was indeed with me, assisting me.

Donna knew more than most, but I didn't tell her everything. She is the primary caregiver for her ninety-six-year-old father, who has a bit of Alzheimer's and her twenty-nine-year-old daughter, who has cerebral palsy. I appreciated every minute she prayed with me on the phone and encouraged me to be strong because there was some divine plan God had for me. As much as I didn't care about this plan, her prayers made me feel better and hooked onto my earlier memories when I wasn't mad at God. When she prayed with me, it reminded me that I had to keep looking ahead, because one way or another, it will all come to an end one day.

After months of crying and begging for help, one long sleepless night, I realized I was calling on a God I had conjured up in my mind from my exposure to various religions, a God that was separate and outside of me; a force I had to appease and beg for mercy to rescue me from my situation. When my pleas went unanswered, I felt abandoned, disappointed, and angry. Then one night through the tears, it dawned on me that I wasn't going to be rescued by this God because that's just not the way it works (well, not in my case anyway).

Somehow I understood that God was more than the limited concept I had in my mind and a force only outside of me. I remembered that God is omnipresent, omnipotent, and omniscient and thought then if God was not only outside of me but also within me, it meant I already had everything I needed to survive this thing that took over my life. I already had courage when I felt tired and didn't want to live and hope when I felt only hopelessness. I already possessed determination when I didn't want to get out of bed every day and self-love to at least give myself a fighting chance by not giving up. Most importantly, I had faith to know that one day, it will all be over.

I understood that the task, however, was to use these characteristics I already possessed to get through my dis-ease. It ultimately was up to me to be courageous, hopeful, and determined, loving myself enough to wake up every day with renewed faith that one day I will be healed.

But, I am a practicing human, and it wasn't always easy to remember this. Who knows, maybe I had to 'lose' God, in a sense, to rediscover the existence of the larger part of me: God.

I was awake more than I was asleep, and a lot of the time, it felt like my thoughts were controlling me rather than the other way around. I had to find a way to busy my mind now that I'd decided against ending my life because every second I contemplated suicide was a waste of energy. I had many hours in a day to think, as all I did was sit. When that got to be too much, I walked from one end of the house to the other. Nothing appealed to me, and if I tried to watch TV as a distraction, it made me more anxious. I couldn't hold my tablet because my arms and fingers hurt, and, because of the pain in my neck, I couldn't rest it on my lap on a pillow to read it.

I browsed some on my phone, which was more comfortable to hold, but nothing kept my attention for very long, as the pain kept reminding me it was always present. The days when I felt utterly depressed, instead of trying to fight it, I allowed myself to sit with it and repeatedly said to myself, *It's only for a moment.* The nights I cried in secret; I kept telling myself, it's only for a moment, which was followed by the thought, *This is a long f*cking moment,* a lot of the times. I also heard my mother's words; this too shall pass, and kept saying it over and over. It was not easy, but it at least kept the unwanted thoughts at bay.

Even though my sisters visited some, and I talked to a couple of people on the phone, no one ever knew my actual pain. When I spoke with anyone, I wanted to enjoy the distraction and forget about the pain for however long the visit or phone conversation lasted. Any overstimulation of my nervous system, from something as simple as talking more than I usually did, caused my body to be nervy for hours after and made my tremors that night much worse. Sometimes during a visit, if I talked more than usual, I felt light-headed, and my heart pounded even more. As much as I appreciated the company, being alone far more often than being in another's company, including William's, meant I had to find a way to keep my mind busy.

I couldn't meditate anymore, as the pain made it difficult to focus. I had to find something to distract my thoughts and found that distraction in music. I love music, especially music with heavy bass, and I listened to anything upbeat to lift my spirits. I listened to old songs and deliberately sang along to keep words in my head. I listened to new songs and tried to learn the lyrics to keep my mind occupied. No matter how my body ached and hurt, there was always one song I couldn't sit out, and I'd have a dance party by myself, which lasted anywhere from twenty seconds to three minutes. Most times, I cried through the movement but forced myself to move anyway. After a few months of having treatments and as the pain decreased bit by bit, I did more exaggerated movements to increase the mobility in my arms and legs.

I had been experiencing pain for so long that it became a significant part of me, and many times at the dinner table, when William asked about my day, I didn't want to talk about it because I started to feel defined by the dis-ease in my body. I didn't want to discuss it with him because that is all we would talk about, and I didn't want the words in my head. I was afraid not only of this thing taking over who I was but of becoming dependent on it.

There were so many things that made me feel bad on so many levels. The fear before we found out what caused my issue. The terror about what would happen to my body and how bad it would get. The loneliness because I didn't want him to see my pain, so I suffered alone in silence—the frustration at myself for allowing my body to get to such a dis-eased state. And of course the pain, tremors and persistent pounding. I felt special and loved when William showed his devotion to me by doing all that he did to help me.

I wanted so badly to feel anything but the mental and physical anguish, and I realized I was becoming addicted to feeling good when he did anything for me. As I started to heal and tried to do more for myself, I had to assert my independence because William had gotten so used to doing everything for me that it had become a part of him also. I had to tread delicately and be careful not to make him feel like I didn't need him anymore. Part of my healing meant enduring pain, and I knew William wanted to protect me from that, but there was no way of getting around it. If I continued to let him do everything for me until he decided it was okay not to, I would have taken that much longer to heal.

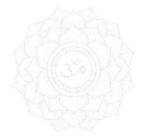

SPIRITUAL JOURNEY

REIKI

fter I graduated from university, I'd been fortunate to work with some great people, doing personally gratifying work as an employment specialist. The government-funded organization I worked with provided job search services to job seekers, and I worked mostly with newcomers to Canada. The one constant in life is change, and after almost eight years working with the organization, my work environment changed and became very stressful. I needed to escape and took the opportunity to go to Trinidad to start the computer training center. The project was the most challenging yet most rewarding thing I'd done in my life to that point. But, sometimes things don't turn out as planned, and when I finally accepted that my brother had different intentions than what he told me, I returned to Canada, jobless and homeless, and what I considered at the time, worse off than when I left.

It was because of the awful feelings of betrayal that I started to question why it seemed that people mistreat each other the way they do. It was difficult for me to understand why my brother went to such lengths to lie, cheat, and manipulate so many people to achieve his goals. Life goes on, and I had to earn a living again and worked for some time in administration until my contract ended. I managed to get a couple of interviews, but deep down, I wasn't very interested in getting those jobs. I thought I missed the freedom that came with working for myself, so I started a home daycare. I enjoyed that too, but still, I felt as though something was missing. There was an intuitive voice inside that said I wanted more, and even though I didn't know what I wanted, I knew I didn't want to work at something just for the sake of money.

When we moved residences, I didn't reopen the home daycare as I decided to take some time to figure out what I wanted to do with my life. William often joked with me, asking, "Hon, what do you want to be when you grow up?" and said I shouldn't worry because I would figure it out someday. I am grateful he didn't put pressure on me, because, one, it gave me more time to spend with Mom during the day, and two, I got to figure out what I wanted to do.

A few days after Mom passed, while I washed dishes at the kitchen sink, I stared out the window at nothing in particular, thinking about nothing. I distinctly heard the word REIKI, and I reflexively looked over each shoulder to see from where the sound had come. I didn't recognize any particular person's voice, but I'd heard it nonetheless. I thought that maybe the fridge had made a weird noise, as it sometimes does, or that perhaps it was someone outside the house, and I didn't think anything more of it.

A few seconds went by, and I continued to wash the dishes, and I heard it a second time: REIKI! Only this time, it sounded more forceful. I instinctively thought, *Okay, in a minute,* not knowing who or what I responded to in my mind. NO! NOW!" was the answer I got. I thought that wherever this is coming from, or whoever it was, they mean business. I took my dish gloves off and went right to my laptop, not knowing what I was going to do. I hadn't heard the word in more than twenty-five years when two aunts had used it in a conversation. Even though I wasn't involved in the discussion, I got the gist of what it was from the explanation.

I didn't have any exposure to Reiki beyond that, but I understood it to be some kind of energy healing. William and I discussed energy healing many times as he had personal experience with it, but we never used the word Reiki. As I powered up my laptop and waited, I still wasn't sure what I would do. When it was ready, I accessed the Internet and googled Reiki classes in my area. A few hits came up, and I clicked the first one. Again the voice, or whatever it was, spoke up, saying, "No, not that one." I wasn't afraid and didn't even think anything was weird with this experience, and I went along with what I heard. I clicked on the second one and browsed the website, learning a little about Reiki.

Reiki is a Japanese word meaning: **Guided Life Force Energy**

I sent an e-mail asking about classes, left my contact information, and closed the laptop, slightly amused. I waited two days for a response, and when nothing came, I called the phone number listed in the contact info on the website and left a voice mail. After another day or so, still, with no response, I went back to my laptop and accessed the list that initially came up. When I clicked on the first option again, I heard, "No!" I quickly closed the website and the laptop and thought, *Okay already. I will be patient.*

My patience was running thin, however, and I complained to William that I was not getting a response though I'd left a message four days ago. He told me to be patient, and he was sure I would get a call soon. Finally, on the fifth day, Michelle, the Reiki Master teacher, called, and we discussed the next upcoming class. I still wasn't sure how Reiki was going to fit into my life and, at best, thought that it was something new to learn.

April sixth was my first class, and I was intrigued by the things I learned. Its teachings resonated with me on a profound level, as I was already trying to live my life by these Reiki principles. I was not always successful, but at least I tried.

1. Just for today, I will give thanks for my many blessings
2. Just for today, I will not worry
3. Just for today, I will not hold on to anger
4. Just for today, I will be honest in all I do
5. Just for today, I will be kind to my neighbor and every living thing

At my first class, there was an attunement ceremony, where the Reiki Master passes down the ability to flow Reiki to the student. Attunement is a very personal experience and different for everyone. We learned that sometimes, after an attunement, a student could experience various physical symptoms, like headaches or a cold. I learned that as the Reiki starts to flow through the energy centers of the body, or chakras, the body tries to rid itself of negative energy, and could manifest itself in different kinds of minor ailments.

My first attunement was April 6, 2017, and on April 7th, I had my first symptom: tingling in my hands. William and I remember it well because we were holding hands (as we frequently do while watching TV) late one evening, and I felt the warm tingling sensation in my hands.

I said to him, "Hon, my hands are tingling!" We joked that maybe my attunement the previous day had something to do with the tingling since the Reiki practitioner uses the hands to flow Reiki, but we didn't give it much thought after that.

The stitch on my left side started within a few days, and it was at my second class that I chatted with a classmate during our lunch break about it. Michelle was in the kitchen while we were in an adjacent room, and I heard her yell, "That is where anger lives, Sherri!"

I was not aware that she'd even heard our conversation about my pain and thought; *Anger is causing my pain?* I didn't pursue it, and after a few more attunements, I became a Reiki Master. The word anger came up again in April of the following year when Tom did his energy testing, and I remembered what Michelle had said a year earlier about anger living where my pain was. In my mind, it was too much of a coincidence to ignore, which is why my journey through dis-ease took the turn it did with Philip.

Another of our neighbors, Irena, had a thriving Reiki practice and spoke mostly to William, as they met each other in the summer months while gardening. We were neighbors for four years, and even though I knew she did energy work, as William told me, the word Reiki never came up. A year after I became a Reiki Master, I met with Irena to talk about Reiki and my symptoms. She said that, when one becomes attuned, the process raises one's vibration, and things like anger, resentment, and other negative emotions have to leave the body. By that point, I'd learned a lot about vibration and the body, in essence being energy, so what she talked about wasn't wholly foreign to me; it still didn't seem that going through this process could bring on such pain. I learned about the possibility of having headaches or colds in our training, but it was difficult to understand something so drastic could occur because of Reiki.

I contacted Michelle to get her take on the likelihood that my body was changing because of Reiki, and she said she'd never heard of someone having such severe symptoms as I had. She shared that she'd had horrid migraines for a year after she became a Reiki Master after never having suffered with headaches.

Am I saying that Reiki was responsible for bringing about my symptoms? I don't know the answer to this question, but I believe that anything is possible. Could it be that I had held on to the anger and fear I experienced as a young child, as well as throughout my life when I witnessed violence and abuse? Could the anger and resentment I felt for my father, while I slowly lost Mom, have added to it and made things worse, contributing to the dis-ease in my body? Could it be that, because I unknowingly harbored anger and resentment for over forty years, my body became ill at ease, and it manifested into a multifaceted physical problem with my spine?

Philip said that the mind may forget, but the body doesn't. Is it possible that the negative emotions (energy) festered in my body until it couldn't take anymore, and my body let me know something was wrong when I had an energy shift because of Reiki?

In the beginning, when I started practicing Reiki, I had a lot of self-doubt because it was all new to me. Even though I knew it was possible, I didn't think I could use Reiki to affect any real change. At the initial stages of my dis-ease, when my pain was a mere discomfort and inconvenience, I practiced self-Reiki and felt the benefits from it, mainly a sense of calm, harmony, and increased energy.

As the pain progressed, however, I started to doubt not only my ability to do Reiki but the Reiki itself. I developed a trust issue and stopped doing it. When I saw the first naturopathic doctor, Dr. Candy, we talked about Reiki, and I told her that I hadn't done it in a long time. She suggested I restart, and, as I did self-Reiki again, I felt better because I slept better. As time passed and my symptoms got worse, though, I stopped again, partly because it was hard to focus on anything because the pain was so bad, and partly because doubt reared its ugly head again. I didn't practice again for a very long time.

I questioned its validity. I was also mad at God, which is the source of this energy, so it all went hand in hand. However, the things I learned about Reiki were always at the back of my mind, trying to come through, and as much as I wanted to ignore it and doubt its legitimacy as a healing modality, I knew in my heart that it works.

In May of 2017, a few weeks after my first symptom, Michelle did a distant Reiki healing for me, which means she did it from her home, and I wasn't even aware she had done it. She first asked my Higher Self's permission to communicate. She then asked questions about the kind of healing I needed and wrote the answers which intuitively came to her. She took pictures of the pages and sent them to me in a text message.

Michelle didn't know much about me when she did my distant Reiki healing because I'd only met her twice before, so when I read her healing message, it confirmed to me the power of Reiki. I knew I had much more to offer; however, the constant self-doubt kept me thinking I was incapable of doing the things I now know we are all capable of doing. My distant Reiki healing not only helped me remember the power of Reiki as a healing tool but also helped me get over my doubt in my abilities. When I read what she sent me, at the time, some of it seemed to apply to me, but when I read it two years later, my experiences became much more relevant and seemed more profound.

- Does her HS have anything more to say?
she has so much to offer but can be her own worst enemy. This is not a roadblock that stop her from progressing it will just create doubt in her abilities. It is so important to create new-ness right now. Stepping outside her comforts. Paying attention to her reactions, and what causes them. Being is a space of awareness. Aware of judgement, aware of behaviours, aware of pre conceived beliefs.

Another thing I found very interesting when I read my healing two years later was my relationship with music and how it contributed to my physical and emotional healing. Maybe I unconsciously remembered what I'd read such a long time ago, but it didn't register when I was looking for a way to create a distraction from thoughts that brought me down. It was so perceptive that Michelle picked up on my love for rhythmic tones because that's precisely the kind of music I listened and danced to when I could ignore the pain for a few minutes or muster up some stamina. I am amazed at her accuracy, two years before I even used music to help heal myself.

I hear drumming and feel the drumming the frequency in my bones. moving and swaying now, HS. she needs movement from music. It will fill her soul. A drum, the rythumy? the beat, Powerful, goddess - fierce.

the vibration of the beat of the tone creates a massive release of hormones in her brain that allows her to "come out of her head" it's the control, the wildness inside screaming to come out, re appear !!

I must explain that Reiki isn't a cure-all for anything. The International Association of Reiki Professionals states,

> It instead assists to create a relaxation response to promote a mind-body state conducive to healing. Curing (in the medical sense) involves alleviating symptoms and treating the physical causes of a health condition. Reiki healing involves spiritual, emotional, and mental unblocking and re-balancing to help get to the root cause of a condition, get back on track and create an optimal environment in which for the body to heal.[26]

While we waited in Dr. Dean's waiting room, I liked to read the informational tidbits regarding the benefits of chiropractic adjustments on his Chiro TV Network. I noticed something about depression and became interested because I suspected I was depressed. As much as I tried everything to stay positive, I was not having a good day—or a couple of weeks for that matter.

As usual, I started my visit with my, "So, I have a question…" opening, with Dr. Dean exclaiming, "WHAT?!" pretending to be surprised. I asked him about the information I saw regarding depression in the waiting room and said I was having a tough time staying positive, no matter how I tried. After explaining how chiropractic adjustments may help depression, he said that even if I didn't feel staying positive worked, it was essential to keep at it. At that point, I felt the tears well up in my eyes because he was telling me to do something I felt was so difficult to do. And even worse, it didn't feel as if it was working.

Dr. Dean has a way of holding your gaze when he explains things, and I didn't want him or William to see my tears. As I listened to him, I did everything I could not to blink or look away. He said that it might not feel like "thinking positive thoughts was working, but the effects of positive thinking are cumulative," which means the more I did it, the better the effects would be. If I kept at it, it would help my healing, even though I didn't feel like anything was happening.

He talked about the feel-good hormones that are released when one is in a positive frame of mind and that these hormones play a significant role in healing. After talking to Dr. Dean about it from a medical perspective, I appreciated more what Michelle had written about music and how it helped me. I remembered that there was a scientific reason why there was a massive release of hormones when I listened to my rhythmic music. The music not only made me feel good because of the beat but also because, during the times when it was too painful to move to the music, I imagined the act of dancing. Most of the time, I imagined myself on a beach somewhere in the Caribbean, which made me feel good, which released more feel-good hormones. I remembered authors such as Bruce Lipton, Ph.D., who spoke about the power of thoughts from a scientific perspective and remembered the impact of positive thoughts on my physical body.

I started doing self-Reiki again in April of 2019 as the pain slowly started to diminish, and as I was able to focus more. Once again, I realized the power of this mode of healing and its positive effect on me mentally, which, in turn, affected my ability to withstand the pain. As much as I didn't practice Reiki amid the emotional and physical pain, I kept the intention somewhere in my thoughts because even that allows Reiki to flow. I held the intention, from a place deep down, that I was going to heal. I kept saying to myself that the end of my pain was somewhere on the horizon, even though it seemed quite the opposite.

We have what we seek. It is there all the time.
And if we give it time, it will make itself known to us.
Thomas Merton (Trappist Monk)

I was also very aware of the power of my words, not only spoken but the thought formations before they become audible words. I've always been mindful of the power of words. For instance, I don't like using the word hate because I think it carries such a heavy negative tone. Sometimes, in casual conversations, William would say, for instance, "I hate the traffic."

I'd respond by saying, "Well, that's a strong word," and we would laugh it off.

Knowing the power of words, I was very aware of the words (thoughts and intentions) that formed in my head or that I used when I wrote in my journal. Even though I wrote about the horrible pain, whenever I ended my journal entries, or a pain got so bad that it held my attention, I would think, *I am healed*, or *thank you for my healing*, as if I was already healed. It was the complete opposite of what my reality was, but I knew I was uttering a self-fulfilling prophecy by saying the words as well as thinking them.

Intentions are also fundamental, and, as I learned through Reiki (as it related to my healing), I had to set the intention to become healthy with my thoughts and words. If anyone ever doubts the power of intention, thoughts, and, by extension, words, one only has to look at Japanese researcher Dr. Masaru Emoto's water-molecule experiment. The premise is that, as humans, we can affect the shape and molecular structure of water just through conscious intention.

The extraordinary life work of Dr. Emoto is documented in the New York Times Bestseller, *The Hidden Messages in Water*. In his book, Dr. Emoto demonstrates how water exposed to loving, benevolent, and compassionate human intention results in aesthetically pleasing physical molecular formations in the water while water exposed to fearful and discordant human intentions results in disconnected, disfigured, and 'unpleasant' physical molecular formations. He did this through Magnetic Resonance Analysis technology and high-speed photographs.[27]

METAPHYSICAL DIS-EASE?

After multiple failed attempts to get help from medical doctors and the likelihood that anger was a potential culprit, I found a book by Evette Rose, called *Metaphysical Anatomy: Your Body is Talking, Are You Listening?* The premise of the book is that traumatic experiences, even those that happen in childhood, can influence and have a direct impact on the disease that may later develop in our bodies. She also talks about ancestral trauma and how it manifests in our present lives. The Merriam-Webster definition of the word metaphysical is "of or relating to the transcendent, extending or lying beyond the limits of ordinary experience or to a reality beyond what is perceptible to the senses."[28]

At first, I went from one symptom to another because I didn't have a proper diagnosis. When we found out what my physical issue was, it was easier to look beyond the physical symptom to understand what potentially caused the dis-ease in my body. I learned some very thought-provoking things, things that seem to fit into the bigger puzzle that was my experience so far. I offer a metaphysical explanation of the most impacted of my spinal vertebrae, as shown on my MRI, thermography scan, and X-rays. According to Metaphysical Anatomy: C1 – "Explore issues related to your living environment, especially during the earliest infancy stages. Was there conflict between your parents? Were you the result of a planned pregnancy?"[29] My mother was nineteen and not married when she became pregnant with me, so it probably is safe to say she didn't plan to have me. I learned that there was physical violence in the home when I was a toddler, and based on my experiences as a young child witnessing it, I can only assume I also observed it at an even younger age than I remember.

C2 – "There is often inflexibility related to how others behave in your environment, which may have a direct impact on you. You often feel that you can't express how you feel about the people around you. You may be stuck in the middle of your parents' conflict."[30] I never felt I could express myself, as Mom always shushed me when I tried to tell my father that his actions were hurtful. I always felt caught in the middle of my parents' marriage, even from a young age. Also, after the fiasco with my brother, I kept everything inside, though I continued to witness his character assassination of me. My mother drilled into my head in the following years, "As long as you know the truth..." I know she meant well, but it was not enough that only I knew the truth. I wanted everyone to know the truth.

C5 – "You feel devalued and often humiliated by what others say to and about you. You feel you cannot restore damage caused to your name and identity as a result of another's bad judgment."[31] Being called a liar and a thief, especially when you try to live by the golden rule, treat others as you want others to treat you, really does a number on your emotional well-being. I felt that I never had a chance to defend myself against the lies.

C6 – "Is activated along with C4, conflict between mother and father, or a parent and sibling. You may want to restore the peace by accepting responsibility for another's mistake. Did your father betray your mother?"[32] A lifetime of conflict! I don't believe I accepted responsibility for another's mistake, but maybe I need to explore this some more.

T2 – "Unresolved anger is surfacing in the way you communicate, as no one is listening to you. Your words do not carry enough power to be respected. As a result, you feel vulnerable to being attacked (verbally) and have no reliable 'tool' with which to defend yourself. You often feel conflicted between two people/desired projects or options within your circumstances."[33] T2 is the one vertebra that felt as if it was literally on fire and caused the most pain in my spine. It took years not to be affected by the things my brother said about me, and I did feel vulnerable. Every time I tried to deal with one lie, another presented itself, and I had to start the process all over again. I was also very conflicted between what my parents and my intuition told me, and my brother's lies.

I also looked up TMJ disorder and was intrigued by the accuracy of what Rose wrote, and how it related to me specifically. A few years before my TMJ disorder diagnosis, two dentists told me that I grind my teeth (most likely in my sleep). During my initial examination, one dentist took pictures of my teeth and showed me the tiny holes in the molars, the size of a pinhead. Neither said there was any cause for concern, so I never followed up until that fateful day in November, when the actual symptom showed itself. According to Rose, the metaphysical reasons for clenching/grinding and TMJ disorder are as follows:

> You have suppressed a great deal of emotions and words. It stems from a time when you were forced to listen to and obey influential people. There may be incidents where this type of trauma has been associated with physical or sexual abuse. You are stewing over old trauma you are too scared to face in your waking life. Unexpressed emotions have transformed into anxiety, tension, and stress. You remember all the words and opinions you were never able to share. You seem to always search for ways to express yourself in a safe way. You were taught to only speak when you are spoken to and were made to feel guilty or bad for speaking up any other time. You may have experienced a significant trauma such as a car accident or traumatic event that shaped your life in more than one way. Grinding (clenching) your teeth is the unconscious mind trying to process and resolve deep emotions.[34]

Was this lady around when I was experiencing all this stuff? I thought. She couldn't be more right, especially about my always searching for ways to express myself. Letter writing has been my go-to safe way to express myself, and I have used it many times over the years. As close as my brother and I were growing up, we had challenges in our relationship when we were young adults, and after one particularly hurtful instance, I wrote him a letter, which I gave him. After I walked away from our business venture, I wrote him another but never sent it because, at the time, I believed just the act of writing my emotions was enough to deal with them.

I also wrote my father a letter during family turmoil and to my sister another time to express my feelings. I wrote my father another letter when Mom lived with William and me, but I never sent it to him. I never regretted it, though, because I truly believed nothing would have come of it. I still have it and who knows, maybe someday he will read it. And of course, there was the letter I left him on the last day I saw Mom alive.

There is too much to write about what Rose says about TMJ disorder. The section is two pages long and has twenty key points to consider. Suffice it to say that this is more than enough evidence to establish a link between my TMJ issues, and my experiences and resulting emotions that brought it on.

I was also curious about Mom's dementia. According to information gathered through hundreds of interviews Ms. Rose conducted for her book about metaphysical anatomy, she wrote this about dementia:

> You feel weak and disempowered when you need to fight your battles. You have been battling with a deep need to control your emotions and are at the final stages of giving up trying to process these conflicting emotions. You may have given up on life as well as on yourself. In most cases, you may be holding on to a lot of guilt toward your children, as you feel like a failure. You have fought a long and hard battle within. You have now had enough of this emotional rollercoaster called life and are disconnected from your inner source of strength. The first key point: giving up is the main key here, why? What happened? What has been a long-standing issue in your life that you could not cope with? [35]

There are some other issues related to childhood, but since Mom didn't talk about negative childhood experiences, I can't say if any of it was relevant to her. When I read this, I had to remind myself, however, not to feel sad for her. I came to understand that these are merely experiences we have as human beings with a specific intention in mind, which is spiritual growth through self-discovery. In the end, it was her experience to have and judge, not mine. When I find I feel sad for her, I joke and say, *Maybe next time,* believing she will have another go at it in another lifetime, if she so chooses.

COINCIDENCE?

thought that, by reading books about spirituality and practicing what I learned, I would better understand spirituality. I now know it's from experiencing things like anger, fear, betrayal, dis-ease, pain, resentment, guilt, regret, and so on, that I gained real understanding, and grew spiritually. So it seems to me that all of these painful emotions, and even the physical pain, play an indispensable role in our lives and are meaningful. As Robert Schwartz says:

> *Life's challenges bring you to the core of your soul's mission, which is always to help you raise your awareness, release judgment, and create an ever wider space of compassion for yourself and others...Each soul creates the life path that offers the best possibility for experiencing the emotions it seeks to understand and make peace with.* [36]

Was everything that happened to me just coincidental? Lexico defines coincidence as a remarkable concurrence of events or circumstances without apparent causal connection.[37]

The probability exists that the series of events resulting in my mis-aligned spine, which caused painful symptoms and problems with my nervous system, was indeed a coincidence. If I view my experiences through a combined, physical, emotional, and spiritual lens, I could say that, just maybe, it was a perfect storm that had been brewing since I was a young child. And which continued to develop as I experienced other traumatic events. If observed, however, through individual physical, emotional, and spiritual perspectives, none of it makes any sense. Maybe Reiki was the catalyst after all the elements were ripe and ready, and the storm hit when my body went through a shift in energy when my vibration changed. How does one prove any of this to be true? If there is a way, I am not aware of it.

I find it hard to believe that there is no rhyme or reason for the dis-ease my body showed, and it was something that just happened to me. The belief that physical disease happens to us just randomly, where we have no control over our health, doesn't resonate with me. I wanted to understand why this happened, and I asked the questions and followed the breadcrumbs to the potential answers. I don't expect people to agree with my perspective because I am not even sure about it myself. My attempt to make sense out of a situation, rather than accept that it just happened, led me to explore other possibilities. I wanted to go beyond what seemed obvious and seek reasons, even though the events leading up to my dis-ease seemed random.

I find this spiritual explanation of synchronicity resonates with my expe-riences more: "Synchronicity is an experience of two or more events which occur in a meaningful manner, but which are causally unrelated. In order to be 'synchronistic,' the events must be related to one another temporally, and the chance that they would occur together by random chance must be very small. When you notice the same coincidence happening more than once, and it begins to take on meaning, then it becomes Synchronicity."[38]

My dis-ease was not supposed to happen to me. After all, I ate well, exercised, meditated, forgave, and had a positive outlook on life, yet there I was with an illness that seemingly just happened out of the blue. I don't think it was out of the blue, though, as my body gave me signs years before the storm broke. I just didn't take the cues because I was unaware. I know this journey of self-awareness has only just begun, and, as my body continues to heal, I know I will understand more. Some people may raise the question of why babies and children get sick, because they may not have the experiences to get them to a dis-eased stage as I proclaim happened to me. As such, they may discount my experiences as having nothing to do with my illness. I question this and other seemingly atro-cious acts that occur on our blue planet, and I still believe there is a reason for everything. I have to because the idea that things happen randomly without reason is too depressing to contemplate. It is, however, up to the questioner to keep an open mind when asking the questions, because the answers exist, and if we take the time to seek, we shall find.

DIVINE PLAN?

Ever since I was a young adult, I have known that someday I would write a book, and for many years I thought, *what could I possibly write about?* I never thought of myself as a writer or did any formal training in writing, or even thought about doing it as a career. A few times over the years, I opened the Word program on my laptop and waited for some kind of inspiration to come, but it never did. However, I never gave up on the idea that one day it would happen.

When I sat in the conference room with the young interns and Dr. James, and I heard his ridiculous diagnosis, something hit me like a ton of bricks. Just under the feeling of absolute despair, there was a profound feeling that I had to share my story so others may learn from it. I knew in my heart and wanted to say, no, doctor, you're wrong! But, knowing that they were the ones with the medical training, not me, I opted to shut up and keep my thoughts to myself.

However, it bothered me in the following days when I thought about how many people were like me, having all sorts of seemingly bizarre physical symptoms and getting diagnosed with a mental illness. I confirmed the feeling that I had to write a book when I remembered that 50 percent of new ER patients get a mental illness diagnosis. All because doctors won't admit they don't know everything and are too quick to slap a vague label on a real medical problem. I know mental illness is real, and I know there are people who (probably) have a somatoform disorder, and I feel for them. But what about the people who don't and doctors tell them that they do!?

I kept thinking about people who may not necessarily have my particular issue, but accept an incorrect diagnosis because (like me at one time) they just want any diagnosis to explain their symptoms. And what about those who potentially do have varying degrees of spinal issues, but because an actual external injury did not cause them, radiologists and doctors consider their results unremarkable, as they did mine?

I had minimal movement in my arms, and my legs were beginning to show the same symptoms, and it was progressing very quickly. There's no doubt that I would have become immobilized and dependent on William until my organs failed because it went unchecked. If we had listened to those doctors, there's no doubt I would have spent the rest of my days drugged up on antidepressants and who knows what other kinds of pharmaceuticals, with their hundred and one potential side effects, to mask the pain. At the same time, the root cause of the dis-ease in my body would have slowly killed me.

I had to share my experience of listening to my gut, my inner voice, my Higher Self because we all have that innate knowing, but we mostly ignore it. I want people to know how important it is to listen to their instincts and offer that there may be more to a physical ailment than meets the eye. And to keep an open mind and at least consider that the dis-ease your body is showing has more to it than just the physical symptoms. I had to share my story and all the twists and turns, the possibilities, probabilities, and coincidences. When I read my Reiki healing from Michelle, another thing stood out to me, and I was in awe because she was unaware of my interest in writing. Just a reminder, this was done eighteen months before we figured out what was wrong.

> 'She writes' - in her head, words flow swirling, poetry - her words are healing. She will heal so many - with words

When the pain was at its worst, and I didn't think I would make it through, something kept saying to me that this was happening for a reason. However, I didn't want to hear it; I didn't want to think about some potential reason having nothing to do with me. I assume it was my Higher Self. However, I was interested only in my pain ending rather than thinking about anything else. When I told my friend Donna about my book, her response gave me shivers. She said, "This was supposed to happen because of your illness. You are supposed to help other people. Not everybody can write a book."

I was thinking the same thing—though not necessarily the part about not everybody being able to write a book—but to hear another person echo my thoughts confirmed that I made the right decision. I know this is how Spirit gives us confirmation when we sometimes ponder something.

It didn't take very long to write, and the words flowed very smoothly. However, I struggled with some of the information I shared regarding my father. The reason, I suppose, is I felt guilty for sharing things that families usually keep secret. I imagine some people saying things like I shouldn't have done this to him, judging me for writing about my experience and seeing it as a betrayal or thinking I am making a big deal about nothing.

I feel very strongly that I had to share my story, which he was involved in, as a supporting character of sorts but just as crucial as ME, the main character. I thought about how hurt my father might be if he were to read my book, and it is not my intention to cause him any pain. There was no other way to convey what I saw, heard, felt, and thought. The essence of the experience couldn't be understood otherwise. I became comfortable with the possibility that maybe it would have no impact whatsoever. Many times over the years, I had conversations with Mom and tried to convince her that he must have at some point thought about how hurtful his behavior was, especially in those moments when he was alone with his thoughts. She told me that she was "doubtful he did," and at some point, I believed her because she was his wife, and (I assumed) knew him better than I did.

PERFECT TIMING

One day, before he did my treatment, Dr. Dean and I talked about the innate intelligence of our bodies to heal, and he mentioned a documentary called HEAL. Sometime later, I found it on YouTube, and as I watched it, I was awe-struck when I heard Dr. Joe Dispenza describe a spinal injury he got in an accident and how he healed himself without surgery. It was so incredible that someone who had such a traumatic injury at so many areas in his spine, healed himself, using only the power of his mind. For a while, after I saw the documentary, I tried to visualize the way Dr. Joe said he did. However, I had a difficult time conceptualizing my healthy spine during the exercise because I had the images of my C-spine MRI and X-rays burned into my brain. Every time I thought of my spine, that's what came to mind.

I managed to focus some, but I didn't think I did that great of a job until Dr. Dean did my second set of X-rays a year after I began having treatments. I didn't think about it at the time, but Dr. Dean said that he was surprised at how quickly I progressed. I joked with him that I certainly didn't feel like it happened quickly. I wondered if any of the visualization I did, contributed in any way to my quicker-than-expected healing. I wasn't all that consistent with my exercises because one, I lost my focus and two because I doubted the possibility that I could do what Dr. Joe had successfully done.

Because I am fascinated by the intelligence of the human body, I am always on a quest for new materials on the subject, and I found another video by Dr. Joe, where he explained more about healing in the quantum field and the science behind it. He talked about our ability to heal ourselves, no matter what the physical condition in our bodies, and how each cell has an innate intelligence and knows what to do to heal.

The recurring theme in his talks was, the power that creates the body heals the body. I began to think again, if Dr. Joe can do it, surely I can do it too. Even he said we are all capable of healing ourselves because we are all born with the same ability to do so.

I started then to consistently take time each day to do a mental rehearsal meditation and imagined my spine healthy, doing things I used to do before like dancing or diving into big waves at the beach. It was again a bit difficult at first to see a healthy spine, but I was determined to do it, and with practice, I am now able to see my spine healthy again.

I recommend the documentary HEAL to anyone who wants to learn about the absolute intelligence and genius of our bodies. After I watched it, I remembered Dr. James' diagnosis that I made up my pain and symptoms. I wonder if I told him what my physical issue is and how I am working toward regaining my health, by having specific chiropractic adjustments and doing mental rehearsals that have a direct impact on my healing, would he tell me that just as I made up my pain, I am also making up my healing. He might be even more discounting about my visualization exercises because he doesn't understand the mind-body connection. The same weekend that I watched the documentary, William, Kathryn, and I took a cousin who was visiting on a tour of the Thousand Islands. Kathryn organized the excursion and invited William and me to go along, mainly because she knew of my love for being near water.

We spent the night at a hotel in the small town of Gananoque, and my tremors were especially violent that night because of the three-hour drive it took to get to our destination. We did the two and a half-hour boat ride the following day, and I thoroughly enjoyed it. The drive home was even longer because we were an extra hour and a half away, and I knew what the night would bring. I thought it best, however, to focus on the lovely time we'd had on the boat and the blue mind I experienced from being on such a massive expanse of water.

While we were away, there was a windstorm at home, and there were a few potted pepper plants that blew over. After we got that cleaned up, William went on to tend to his vegetable garden and flowers around the house. My cousin and I stood on the porch and watched William as he watered the flowers, and I began to share with her some of my experiences over the last few years. Not too long into our conversation, I started to feel a bit light-headed and chalked it up to the overexertion of the previous two days. As my light-headedness got worse, I stopped our conversation and headed inside.

Then something happened! I felt an erratic flutter in my solar plexus, and it terrified me because, as much as I'd had the beating sensation in this area for so long, it felt nothing like this. I didn't think it was my heart but wondered if it was possible because I knew women showed symptoms differently than men do.

After explaining what I'd felt, I held my cousin's hand against my solar plexus and asked if she could feel the flutter, and she said she did. I thought I'd caused my body more stress by talking about the past, and I was sure it affected me. I knew the physical signs. I said, "See! This is what happens when I talk about it," while her hand was on my stomach, feeling the erratic beat. Her phone rang, and I left the TV room where we were, went to the living room a few feet away, and sat down. I didn't want the drama of scaring her if I collapsed.

I'd asked her to feel the fluttering because I didn't know what caused the sensation; I wanted someone to know the symptom I had preceding my passing. I was sure my time had come, and I was ready, oh so ready, and made peace with everything! I sat on the sofa, quietly, waiting for whatever happened next.

In the few minutes this thing fluttered, I felt absolute peace and love. I thought about William, who was outside watering the flowers, oblivious to what was happening, and I felt such love and appreciation for him. My heart felt like it would overflow with gratitude. Then my thoughts shifted to the other love I believed I was heading toward; the love of my mother! I felt almost as euphoric as I did when I'd laid on her tummy in her room that day. I breathed through it and waited, and the flutter slowly calmed down and eventually disappeared.

When I realized I wasn't going to die from this weird thing, I thought about my sessions with Philip, as well as all the emotions I'd convinced myself I'd dealt with while writing. I wondered if I was still holding on to negative emotions. I had started taking the OTC sleep aids only on the nights I had treatments because they began to mess with my digestive system again, so I didn't take one on this particular night.

I went to bed, expecting the same routine of dozing off to sleep only to be roused by the tremors. As my body relaxed, I felt as if I was still on the boat, and it was very soothing like I was gently rocking but without the vibration or noise of the boat engine. I felt my body drop into relaxation and got a bit anxious because I knew what usually followed. I waited for the infernal tremors.

THERE WERE NONE!

I fell asleep on my own and only realized this when I opened my eyes at 4:42 a.m. I went to the bathroom, got back into bed, and fell asleep again. No tremors. For over two years, I'd suffered from this hideous sensation that plagued me every night, and I wondered what the heck had happened. I thought maybe the rocking sensation superseded the tremors because my body felt as though it were still moving, so it didn't tremor. I told my cousin the following morning, but not William, because I wasn't sure what had happened and I didn't want to get his hopes up, or mine for that matter.

During the day, I shared more of my story with my cousin, and she patiently listened to my endless chatter and expressed her surprise at the things I told her about her aunt's experience. She said she remembered the videos of Mom that my father shared with family, and she now understood why Mom had a certain look in her eyes. I didn't have the flutter during our conversation, so I thought that maybe I was okay.

I had my biweekly treatment with Dr. Dean later that evening. I expected the typical aftereffects of worse than usual tremors because my nervous system got aggravated on account of the treatment. I went to bed, as usual, that night. As my head hit the pillow, I remembered I hadn't taken a sleep aid, but I was so tired and drained, and I didn't want to bother William and thought I would play it by ear; If the tremors came on, I'd ask him to get it for me. I was also curious if not having tremors the night before was a one-off and wanted to see what would happen, especially on the night of my treatment.

As usual, I put my timed meditation music on and waited for the dreadful vibrating sensation somewhere in my body. Again, THERE WAS NONE! It wasn't very long after that I dozed off without even a tiny vibration! I woke up at 6:12 a.m. when I heard William moving about to get ready for work. For someone like me, who's pretty good at expressing myself with written words, there are none to communicate how I felt when I realized the tremors were potentially over and done with, and my body could now fall off to sleep on its own.

My cousin and I talked about it the next day, and we thought that the flutter I felt was probably a release of the last bit of negative energy I had in me. Sharing with William, Philip, and Kathryn, and through my writing, all had a part to play in my healing. My experience with my cousin was even more remarkable because our families had lost touch for over twenty years, and it happened by coincidence that she came to spend time at my home. She said she finally accepted Kathryn's invitation to visit after being harassed weekly, and hadn't even been sure she would be successful in getting her visa because the process is usually a long and unpredictable one. She got through quite easily when others who had applied before she did were not successful.

William tried to convince me to go back to Trinidad with my cousin so that I would have company for the trip. He kept insisting that I needed to get away from everything for a while, even if it was only for a couple of weeks. He believed that being stuck in the house for almost two years had taken an emotional toll and that reconnecting with family and friends again would have a positive effect on my healing. I fought him on the idea because I didn't want to miss so many treatments.

He brought up the idea at one of my treatments with Dr. Dean, and he agreed with William. I expressed my concern about missing treatments and the six-hour flight. I was also worried that if I got the tremors again, I wouldn't be in my own space and would be uncomfortable. Sometimes at home, I'd go downstairs and walk around or just sit when the tremors wouldn't let me sleep. I didn't want anyone to worry about me if things went awry. Every time I saw Dr. Dean, he and William tried to convince me of the benefits of a break. When I asked if I would regress if I missed treatments, he explained, with a cautionary tone, "Well, yeah a bit, but the benefits of the emotional connections you would have and being back home would far outweigh any regression."

I thought about it, but I'd had these awful tremors for so long that the mere idea of having them again, so far away from home, made me very anxious. I didn't have to debate with myself for much longer about going or not going, though, because William surprised me with a ticket to Trinidad for my fifty-first birthday. I was excited but apprehensive because part of me did want to get away for a while. Dealing with the roller-coaster rides with doctors, and the gradual decline of my physical, emotional, and mental health took everything I had, and I wanted to escape it for a while. The idea of not having treatments and the aftereffects was tempting, and my excitement about my impending trip finally surpassed my worry.

The plane ride was longer and more uncomfortable than I'd remembered. Still, I kept thinking about the beaches I would soon be on and distracted myself with visions of reconnecting with friends and family I hadn't seen in almost five years—some for more than twenty years.

My first night in Trinidad was pure hell! The tremors were back, and they were relentless! They were so bad that they felt violent. Oh, how I wanted my bed and my own space. I watched as the minutes and hours went by. As much as it felt like time was flying by, it also felt as if it had slowed down. I had these moments at home when the tremors wouldn't let me sleep, and when I checked the time, I couldn't believe only an hour had passed, but it felt like the tremors were ongoing for much longer. I didn't sleep one wink, not only because of the tremors but also because I had a difficult time getting used to my new environment—the bed, the split unit A/C I couldn't adjust, and the new noises.

Was it too good to be true? I didn't have tremors for a couple of weeks, and here they were again. I fought off the depressing thoughts in the solitude of my room, not wanting to alarm my host. I couldn't help but question if my luck had run out and why. I'd had a taste of sleeping without this dreadful sensation, and here it was again, and it was frightening. I can only assume that the long day of getting ready for my flight, the actual journey, the vibration of the plane, sitting for over six hours, and now my new environment caused the perfect storm for my tremors again. I took sleep aids with me just in case, and even though I took one, it was no use. I couldn't bear the thought that the next fifteen days of my vacation would be like this.

I had many hours that night to think about why this was happening to me again. I didn't have tremors after I had the experience with my cousin, and I wondered if maybe there was an emotional component to those particular tremors that stopped.

A light bulb went off! My nervous system may have been physically overstimulated, which could have potentially caused the tremors to return. It was then that I realized there is a strong possibility, there was an emotional and a physical trigger that caused these tremors I'd been experiencing for so long. That they started up again and they were so bad the night I got to Trinidad, could have been because of the physical overstimulation. My body felt nervy when I finally made it to bed after the long day, and I am sure that, because my nervous system was physically overstimulated, this is what caused the tremors to start again. If my vagus and other nerves are affected because of the spinal compression, it makes sense that anything (in this case, the long flight and vibration of the plane) that irritated the nerve or nerves would result in the tremors. My nervous system was on overload, and it was not happy!

Fortunately, my vacation turned out to be fantastic! Spending time with family fed my soul, and I fed my belly with local dishes that tasted even more delicious because I didn't cook them. The warm sunny weather had a different effect on my body and mind than the summer I left in Canada. Spending time at my favorite beach gave me a sense of peace and serenity I often long for, and I had only two nights of slight tremors, which I was able to get past without sleep aids.

One of the nights I got the tremors, we'd had a long drive to the beach house, and it was very tiring. The other night I got them, I'd frolicked in rough waters during the day and got pounded by some big waves. I had very little pain because I hadn't had treatments, and whatever pain I did have, resulted from sleeping on six different beds while visiting family. My body was in different positions, and even though the change was small, it still affected me. I was cautious to stay physically and emotionally calm before going to bed relatively early. William and Dr. Dean were right;

the benefits of taking a break from my life far overshadowed whatever regression I would have by missing treatments.

My parents used to say to us as children, "Wait! After joy is sorrow!" when we got too rowdy and could potentially hurt ourselves when we didn't heed their multiple warnings. As an adult, I've always thought it was a warped way to think that after one has a good time, something terrible will always follow. In this, they were right!

When I resumed treatments after my wonderful vacation, it was nothing short of sorrow! The headaches and body pain were off the charts, and so were the tremors and pounding in my body. It took over two weeks to get back to my normal level of pain I'd had before my vacation. Dr. Dean ramped up the intensity of my treatments, and it resulted in even worse tremors (physical overstimulation). Some nights, I was up for six hours after going to bed because I refused to use pharmaceutical sleep aids again, and the OTC ones didn't work. I learned that sometimes if I shook my legs when the tremors started, they would stop for a few minutes before it happened again. I would do this multiple times and was able to fall off to sleep during one of the moments in between the tremors.

I wasn't always that lucky, and there were some nights the tremors got so bad, shaking my legs wasn't enough, and I had to get up and walk around, to 'reset' my body. When I first tried to get off the lorazepam, I had tried Bach's Rescue Night, an herbal sleep aid before bed but it didn't help, because as soon as I started to doze, the tremors would come on and wake me and I couldn't go back to sleep. Not wanting to use pharmaceutical sleep aids, one night, out of pure desperation, I waited for the tremors to start, and as soon as I felt them, took the Rescue Night, and somehow it worked. It seemed as though if I let my body get to a relaxed state on its own, then took the Rescue Night just as the tremors started; it gave me that extra edge I needed to fall asleep. If I didn't time it just right, however, I would be up for hours because I missed the window, and even if I took an additional sleep aid, it didn't work.

On an interesting note: Six months after my crazy flutter experience, I was having a casual conversation with someone familiar with how energy works. We were discussing my infernal tremors and the potential emotional connection to them. I expressed how the sensation is so unnerving, and I just wished it would stop. He pointed out that the energy of illness and the energy of health, are two different energies potentially existing in my body, fighting for space and that this fight can manifest as physical tremors. He suggested that just like I'd had treatments to allevi- ate the negative physical energy (the physical pain) in my body, and it took time, getting rid of other negative energy (emotional) also wouldn't happen overnight. I had another AHA moment and remembered Irena's explanation about how my body changed when I started doing Reiki. It's a perspective I hadn't thought of, but it is rather amusing).

IMPROVEMENT!

In March of 2019, I went out for the first time in almost two years and attended a family event. When Kathryn invited me to the surprise birthday party, she joked that I should be prepared for hugs because I was still very sore to the slightest touch. I had not seen my family in such a long time, and one of my uncles, who is known for not saying much, held me by my arms and squeezed them so tightly, I almost yelled out in pain. It took everything not to pull away from him because I couldn't explain at the time why I hurt so much. He looked me square in my eyes and asked, "Are you happy?" I said, yes, I was, and he responded, "Good!"

Even though I texted him the following day to say thank you, he would never know how much I appreciated his hug and concern for my happiness. I got an even tighter hug from my cousin, and she squeezed me so hard, I heard my neck snap. It was a sound I'd heard more times than I can count as I started moving my arms and neck again. It was a fun night, but I couldn't stay until the end because it was my first outing in almost two years, and it took a lot out of me physically and emotionally.

Everything I did became a form of therapy; every movement caused agonizing pain, but I knew if I didn't work through it, I would never heal. Every dish I held to wash hurt my fingers, every time I stretched to get something from or put something into a cupboard, my sides hurt. Every vegetable I cut to make a meal caused agonizing pain in my arms and neck, but I knew it was the only way to regain the use of my arms. The more I did these natural movements, the more my pain eased, and my flexibility improved. Still, the changes were so minor, literally millimeters over months, and if I didn't pay attention, I would have missed my progress and felt as though I was not healing.

There is qualitative improvement in how I now move my body, compared to how I was at my worst when I could barely lift my arms a few inches from my sides. I've had adjustments now for twenty-two months, and I have come a long way. I am now able to do things I was not capable of before because of the pain and limited movement caused by the muscle atrophy in my arms and neck.

I have moments of some or worse pain, and I focus on the moments I feel relief and remind myself that, even though I have pain, I am getting better, and one day soon, I will be pain-free. I have about 50 percent lateral movement in my left arm and about 70 percent in my right. I can now raise my arms in front of me about 90 percent, but with some pain. I've had to get quite creative in how I accomplish tasks because I know the only way to get full movement again is to go through the motion, even if it causes more pain.

My mantra has become, *If it hurts, it needs to heal,* to brainwash myself into doing things even when the result is even more pain. I use an at-home ultrasound device to help heal the muscles and ligaments in my arms, and I do small exercises to increase my range of motion incrementally. Sometimes I get the pulling sensation under my left foot, and it's quite jolting because it happens when I least expect it. Dr. Dean advised me to use a golf ball, and while resting the sole of my foot on it, roll it around under my foot to loosen up the muscles and ligaments. It helps, and the ease sometimes lasts for days. I now walk for forty minutes on my treadmill, five times a week. Granted, I am not able, just yet, to do my three to four and a half miles a day at 3.8 to 4 mph; instead, I now walk at a leisurely 2.3 mph. I know in my heart that if I hadn't kept moving on my treadmill throughout my ordeal, things would not have turned out so well for me.

I now make meals a few times a week, though I'm still unable to cut hard vegetables like a sweet potato or squash, but I manage (if I get help) to cut it to a manageable size. I mostly dress myself, and I now wear my t-shirts instead of William's—his were easier to put on. Most times, I put my tank top on over my head instead of pulling it on like pants from my legs up and wiggling into it, but I still need a bit of help with tighter tops and jackets that aren't very stretchy. Even though I still struggle with washing my hair, I no longer bend over to complete the task, and it doesn't cause debilitating pain in my sides like before. I consider the minimal pain to be therapy and push through it.

I went from needing William's assistance to put my hair up, to bending over to do it myself, to now mostly being able to put it up the usual way. I no longer look like I'm trying to start a funky new hair trend with my hair sitting on top and to the front of my head. I take care of all my hygiene needs, including drying my hair.

I started driving again, able to do only short outings every few days because using the muscles required for driving caused more pain in my neck, arms, and sides. Sometimes I get a bit skittish if I hear a car horn honk for more than a second. It evokes the memory of when I was on the wrong side of the road, and my fellow road users cussed me out while honking their horns. I do some household chores and found out the hard way that mopping the traditional way results in severe pain, so I stand on a wet cloth and dance while I drag my feet to clean the floors.

The tingling in my hands has mostly subsided, and I don't have a warm sensation like before. My itchy legs are better, and I don't scratch the top layer of my skin off when I sleep. I still have the itchiness at times, but not like I did before. This particular improvement confirms for me the relationship between spinal compression and its effects, like a seemingly weird symptom such as itchy legs. My weight has stabilized at 123 pounds, and my digestive system has improved since I stopped taking OTC sleep aids. Depending on the intensity of my treatment, the sensitivity on my back, neck, and arms, flare up, but I no longer have to shield myself from clothes or my favorite silk duvet. I also get a tightening sensation in my sides and legs after treatment, and it's not very comfortable, but at least it's tolerable.

I learned that emotional overstimulation doesn't necessarily have to be negative either. Once, we stayed up until 2:00 a.m., spending time with guests who visited, and I laughed until my cheekbones hurt. We had a great time and ate the most delicious chocolate cake with ice cream at 11:00 p.m. I realized I'd pushed myself too much when, in one of those moments of frenzied laughter, I felt light-headed, and my solar plexus felt as if it would explode. I quickly said, "I'm tapping out," and by the time I made it to bed, I couldn't relax because of the pounding in my body. An hour and a half later, I took a sleep aid, but it didn't help. The good news is that I didn't have tremors because I didn't even get to the dozing-off stage of sleep that night.

Even though I can quantify my improvement, I am stuck in a place where I have to be cautious about how much I do, both physically and emotionally. The pounding still bothers me, and it sometimes affects my ability to even get to the point of dozing off to sleep. Sometimes, if I sit still after climbing the stairs, for instance, I can feel my eyeballs pulse with every beat of my heart, and I see the vibration. If I push myself physically too much and cause pain, it makes the pounding worse; it then takes days for my nervous system to calm down.

I wanted to confirm for my peace of mind that the ramped-up treatments were responsible for the increased tremors and pounding, so I took a day off from my Thursday treatment. A couple of days before my scheduled treatment the following Monday, I was finally able to fall asleep naturally because I got past the minimal pounding with no tremors. My nervous system was able to calm down because there was some extra time between treatments. We decided to reduce my treatments to once a week and increase the intensity because doing it twice a week didn't give my body enough time to recuperate.

Dr. Dean said maybe the increased intensity would one day cause the spine to move just enough to take the pressure off the nerve and result in the tremors and pounding ending. I so look forward to the day my body can feel relaxed because the constant pounding that gets worse with physical or emotional overstimulation is not fun.

The pain is consistent, but so is the improvement! After I've had a treatment, the pain is always in different areas with varying intensities. At times I can putter in the kitchen and help with dinner, and others, all I can do is sit as soon as I get home from my treatment. Mornings continue to be the worst time of the day because, upon waking, my muscles (which were dormant for a few hours) hurt like the dickens, and the first movements of the day almost bring tears to my eyes.

I feel this way not only because of the pain but from the frustration of having started my day, feeling so rotten. In these moments, I give thanks for my healing and remind myself it was much worse two years ago. There is an instant change in my attitude, and I have good days despite everything.

After a few months of using the natural sleep aid and having some control over the tremors to get some sleep, it (like the pharmaceuticals and OTC sleep aids) also started to lose its effect; I was back at square one again. I would be up for four or five hours trying to fall asleep, some nights doing all I could not to become depressed. I felt as though I had made one step forward and two steps backward. Over the last three years, when the pain was as its worst, and I couldn't get to sleep, I listened to meditation music on YouTube to try to distract myself from my thoughts. When the Rescue Night and shaking my legs failed to stop the tremors, I thought I would try another meditation to relax, but I needed something more than music. I searched for a guided meditation and found one by Jason Stephenson called *Heal Your Body, Mind Whilst You Sleep*. It was a little over two hours long, and I figured if nothing else, at least my mind would be preoccupied listening to words.

He has a very soothing voice, and his Australian accent made what he said even more engaging. As I listened to his instructions, which was to focus on the breath and different areas of the body, he mentioned something called Yoga Nidra. He explained that "Yoga Nidra takes you to a place between restfulness and sleep…where the mind is as calm as can be while still (being) conscious. It's also here that you are at your most powerful because it is in this state, the barriers between your conscious and subconscious mind, are at their weakest."[39] As I listened to the meditation, I was very aware of my surroundings, but at the same time, I felt the most relaxed I had ever felt doing a meditation.

I felt the tremors come on, but they lasted only for a few seconds and stopped. Not long after, I dozed off because I felt the pounding increase, which usually happens as I doze, but I was able to get past the sensation to have a full night sleep; I only realized this when the sun lit up the room in the morning. When I became more awake, I thought I must have been so tired from almost four weeks of little sleep that my body finally caved in a fell asleep. My sleep felt different, though, more restorative than when I used sleep aids. I couldn't remember the last time I felt so good, and I had a great day because my overall general feeling of well-being was nothing short of amazing. The sleep was even better than those times I fell asleep naturally after my flutter experience when the tremors stopped.

The following night, I went to bed a bit apprehensive thinking the night before must have been a fluke. Not very long into the meditation, I fell asleep again, feeling not even a tiny vibration in my body. The pounding was so minimal I think I fell asleep around fifteen minutes or so into the meditation. Night three, same thing! I dozed off at some point in the meditation, and I knew this because I couldn't remember some parts of it the next day. I knew when it was over because I removed my headphones and went right to sleep. I couldn't believe this was happening and wanted to understand why this Yoga Nidra had such a different result than so many other kinds of meditations I had done over the last decade.

Yoga Nidra translated from Sanskrit, means Yogic Sleep. Yoga Nidra is much like hypnosis; "however, the Nidra practitioner is encouraged to stay awake and alert. This deeply relaxed state is the parasympathetic nervous system (PNS) in full force. The PNS is the relaxation response, and it's crucial for healing. The body can't begin to repair and restore itself, to heal, until we move out of the stress response, which is the sympathetic nervous system (SNS), and into the parasympathetic nervous system."[40]

Wikipedia says that "Yoga Nidra allows a state of consciousness between waking and sleeping, and there is evidence that Yoga Nidra helps relieve stress. An ancient technique from India, it has now spread worldwide and is also being applied by the US Army to assist soldiers in recovering from post-traumatic stress disorder."[41]

I think I fell asleep without the tremors doing Yoga Nidra because, even though I was in a relaxed state, I was still conscious. Maybe my body (or brain) didn't know it was relaxed and possibly on the verge of sleep, so it didn't tremor. Talk about tricking the brain, but without antianxiety meds!

I did this meditation consistently for a few weeks, sometimes falling asleep a few minutes into it and sometimes intermittently waking and falling back to sleep over the two hours. I'm not cured of the tremors just yet, though. One Sunday afternoon, I tried to nap (without the meditation), and I couldn't because they came on as soon as I dozed off. The tremors are also more intense on the nights after I have a treatment or any overstimulation of my nervous system, so it takes longer to get past them because I have to shift my body to stop them. Is this the answer to healing my over-active sympathetic nervous system that has been on alert practically all of my life, and especially over the last nine years? I can only hope and time will tell how it will all play out. Still, I can fall asleep without sleep aids, and I hold on to the hope that because my body is naturally getting into the parasympathetic state, my healing will now happen a lot faster. It's just a matter of time before the tremors and pounding will be a long-forgotten distant memory.

I had a second spinal thermography scan done nineteen months after the initial one, and I was surprised that C2 showed a red bar when it didn't show on the first scan. Dr. Dean reminded me that it is a snapshot of what is happening in the spine on a given day, and the results will depend on what kind of activity one does. Earlier in the day, Keith Urban, the vacuum and I had a dance party, while I vacuumed, and I might have overdone it a bit, especially when the song *The Fighter* (which I replayed a few times) played. I must have aggravated my spine at C2, and so the muscles, tendons, ligaments that connect to it.

In comparison, I now have a lot of blues, and according to Dr. Dean, it means we're turning the volume down and getting better clarity of signals as a whole coming through those areas. The smaller the bars are, the closer I am to the next level of color on the scale, so the smaller the blue bar, the closer I get to the green bar. The smaller the red bar, the closer I get to the blue bar, and so on. There are noticeable differences in my follow-up scan, which shows consistent improvement in my spine. For those who are critical of chiropractic, discounting this form of healing for whatever reason is senseless. At best, it helps a patient to heal, and at its worst, if even it is seen as a placebo, at least there are no potential unwanted side effects like the ones pharmaceuticals can cause.

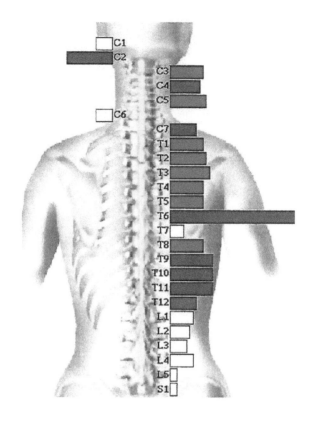

Spinal Thermography

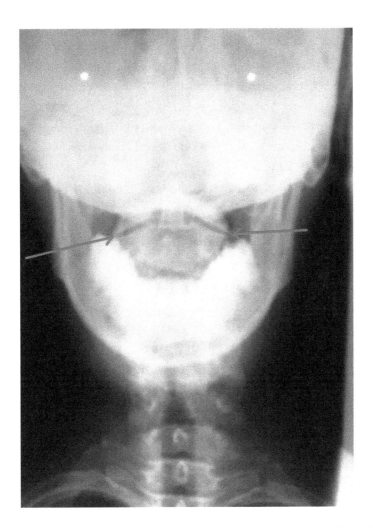

I also did another APOM X-ray to check on the progress of my C1/
C2 vertebrae. There is a definite and significant difference between this
one and the other I took at my initial consultation in 2018. The space
on the left side has opened up even though it may seem subtle. Dr. Dean
reminded me that we are dealing with fractions of millimeters when
it comes to the movement of the spine. Because the pain in my arms,
fingers, and sides is decreasing and I am slowly regaining range of motion
in my arms, this is proof that I am indeed healing.

When I saw Dr. Michelle for my menopausal issues, she recommended pelvic floor physiotherapy. I was amused because I didn't think one could have physiotherapy for their pelvic floor. When I started to feel better, I met with Laura, the physiotherapist. When she did my assessment, she found that my pelvic floor muscles, as well as the muscles around my diaphragm, more so on my left side, were tight. She explained that many people hold stress in their pelvic floor as well as the diaphragm, by unconsciously holding in or tightening these muscles. She said it is a way of protecting our internal organs (and especially the reproductive organs for women) from perceived threats. When we are stressed, we also don't breathe fully and extend our breath, and this can potentially cause issues in the diaphragm.

I found it interesting, too, when she said that holding in the pelvic floor muscles can lead to constipation (for obvious reasons). I knew I was tightening up my pelvic floor muscles, but I wasn't aware of how much I did it until I tried to relax them. When I became more conscious of it, I realized that I was also doing the same with my stomach muscles. I knew I did it when I was scared or stressed about something, but I didn't think I did it under 'normal' circumstances. Both Laura and Dr. Dean agreed that the constant tightening up of these (and associated) muscles most likely caused the stitch in my sides and under my last set of ribs.

It makes sense because the diaphragm is a sheet of muscle that runs diagonally at the bottom of the thoracic cavity. Whether my misaligned pelvis caused the issue or the tightening caused my spine to move is a toss-up. Stress, however, seems to be the common denominator, and it's taking a lot of conscious effort to relax both these muscles. It amazes me how unaware you can be that you are doing something until you try to stop doing it! The last piece of the puzzle, and now it all makes sense.

Laura recommended the happy baby yoga pose, along with other exercises to help relax my pelvic floor and to get the muscles connected to my pelvis moving properly again. She also advised me to be mindful of my breathing, to fill my lungs, and expand my diaphragm fully as if sending my breath all the way through. We are also working on getting my arms moving again because I've reached the limits of what I can do on my own.

One of the questions on the form I filled out before my initial visit asked if I believed I would heal. I brought it up in my session with Laura, and we talked about why they ask this particular question. She said that many people might need her help to get healthy again, but if they answered that they didn't believe they would regain their health, she got a sense of the mindset of the patient and what to expect. She said that she could do all the physio in the world with a patient, but if they didn't believe they will be healthy again, her work would all be in vain. We agreed that healing begins in the mind, and *believing* that you will be healed, is half the work.

I have yet to do a follow-up MRI of my C-spine because I am curious about my C6/C7 vertebrae and what effects the adjustments have had on this area of my spine. When my fingers no longer hurt and tingle and my arms are pain-free and fully functional, I will take that as a sign that all is well and I will have it done. Every day I heal a little, and I know one day soon, I would look back on the last three years of my life and say *WOW!*

IT'S ALL ABOUT PERSPECTIVE!

As I started to feel better, I began to analyze and put my experience into perspective. I considered the three options available to me: One, I could try to forget my horrible experiences because they were so painful. Two, I could stay angry at the seemingly hurtful things that happened. Or three, I could make something good and positive come out of my experiences, despite how painful they were. I realized if I chose option one, I would most likely end up in the same place maybe at a later stage in life, less able to endure the consequences because the mind may forget, but the body doesn't. I believe some other experience or dis-ease would have presented itself to offer me the opportunity to learn whatever lessons my soul wanted to learn. Option two would most likely end just as horribly as I've learned anger and other negative emotions (whether you are aware of them or not) fester in the body and eventually manifest as dis-ease. Option three was my only choice, and I decided to not only learn from my experiences but also to potentially help others understand theirs.

Writing this book has also been a form of therapy for me. When I started to write about my childhood experiences and how I dealt with it in therapy with Philip, I realized I still had some residual emotions. As I wrote and reread, my body trembled and tensed up, especially my stomach area, but I noticed that the more I read and edited, the more my body relaxed. It was as if the anger and fear were peeling away, layer by layer, every time I read what I wrote. There came the point where I no longer had the intense physical symptoms I did when I first started writing. I thought that, after dealing with it in therapy, I was okay, but my body told me differently. I then understood that healing, whether it is physical, psychological, or emotional, is a process, and it takes time.

More importantly, I realized that it is through the process that I learned more about myself and why I think, feel, and react to situations the way I do. I am still learning, but my awareness has expanded, as one question led to an answer, which led to another question, which led to another explanation and so on. I've learned that even though I had these thoughts and experiences, and they helped me to understand myself better, they do not define me, and they are not who I am. They are just things. One could say, parts of me that make up my humanness. As important and probably necessary as they were, I am more than *just* my experiences.

The act of writing and sharing my experiences has been a therapeutic one, and as I wrote, I felt an acceptance for everything sink into my being. Also, I found that as I wrote, I seemed to work things out in my head, as thoughts I hadn't considered before appeared. For instance, I found it very interesting that for most of my life, from when I was around five, whenever I got scared, I had the same pounding sensation in my solar plexus and a tightening in my abdomen when my body vibrated to the point where it felt locked up. I felt the same way when I visited Mom and experienced fear and anxiety because of the way my father treated me. These are exactly the symptoms I have now and am trying to heal. After giving up Mom because of the emotional toll it took on me, I seemed to be doing okay because the cause of those fears no longer existed, or so I thought. It was a mere three weeks after she transitioned that my symptoms started to show.

Like Tom said, it seems as though I'm stuck in the fight or flight response, but he was only half right when he thought it was because of the pain I'd had for a year. It went far beyond that one year and included every other experience that caused my heart to pound and my body to tremble and tense up. I am in perpetual awe of the resilience of my body and how it was able to function for over forty years before showing its dis-ease. I have to convince my body now to relax since there is nothing to run away from or fight.

The other thing I find interesting is that the 'voice-lessness' that came with the kind of dementia Mom had was very much how she felt. She didn't think her feelings and opinions mattered, and many times I wonder if she ever felt validated in any way. I think of her sometimes when after we have dinner, William thanks me for the meal and says how delicious it was, sometimes even texting me from work the next day to say he enjoyed his leftovers. Ten years later, he still thanks me when I do the laundry or other household chores. I remember the times my father told Mom she "had nothing to study but cooking and cleaning," with a tone that was not loving or appreciative but rather reproachful and condescending.

Writing this book also saved my sanity because as I started to feel better, I got very restless. I was in a constant battle between feeling anxious and convincing myself that I was doing the vital work of healing. I felt like I was wasting my life away, doing nothing for many hours a day. Not being able to put on a coat by myself in the winter, and, when the weather got nicer, being unable to drive, I felt like a prisoner at home. I was never much for watching TV, and there was only so much I could stand to read about world events, as those were sometimes depressing. Writing gave me something to do and kept me occupied while I healed.

As I wrote, I wondered if all of this is part of the perfection of life because, if I hadn't had all the experiences I did, which I believe resulted in my body becoming dis-eased, I would not have had any of the experiences which followed. My lifelong dream of writing a book may never have happened because I would have no subject matter. If I had been working and carrying on, as usual, I am also sure I wouldn't have had the time to write like I did while I was healing because there was nothing to do but write. Sometimes I even wonder about my desire to write a book; where did that come from, and was it part of my soul's plan? Was it my inner voice reminding me over the years about my plan?

I even thought about my experience at the kitchen sink when I heard the word Reiki; was that also my consciousness starting me on the path that led to this book? The trail of events and experiences which led to this book may be all the evidence I need, as it all dovetailed perfectly.

I believe it's all about perspective, and I choose to appreciate all that happened to me as the natural perfection of the universe and be grateful for all I have learned. As I pondered this for a couple of days, I opened my e-mail and got this 'note from the universe,' which said:

*How adventurous would life be, Sherri, if you were 'challenge free?'
If you had the perfect body, perfect self-esteem, everyone adored you,
and you won the lottery every Sunday? NOT! Now, what if, painful as
they may temporarily be, you could choose a life during which challenges
might arise whenever your thinking needed expansion, on the sole condition that every one of them could be overcome no matter how daunting
they may first seem? Everything makes you more!* [42]

OK, it might be wonderful to have all these things and win the lottery
every Sunday, but maybe all that perfection would get boring after a
while. How else would we grow if we didn't have life challenges?

When Kathryn suggested I keep a journal of my symptoms, it started
as a way to document the progress of my dis-ease, but journaling became
a form of therapy in its own right. What I felt I couldn't talk to William
or anyone else about, I was able to let the feelings and emotions out
through writing. William suggested I share my journal with readers, and I
contemplate it, going back and forth because it exposes some of my most
private thoughts. I do believe it's important for others who are having a
tough time, whether emotionally or with a medical ailment, to know that
it's natural and okay to feel despondent, emotionally drained, or whatever
else they feel. There were up days I wished would last forever, and down
days when I wanted to give up. Maybe sometime in the future, I will
share it because, even as I write, I am still healing and consider myself a
work in progress.

Regarding my relationship with my family, I decided to withdraw
myself because I will not socialize with my father or brother, knowing
what I know. There was no indication that either of them was going to
change the way they behaved toward me, and I will not be in a relationship with either of them and allow the behavior to continue. In the book
Everything is Here to Help You, I learned that "there is no spiritual benefit
for staying in an environment as someone's mental, physical, or energetic
punching bag."[43]

Even though I am self-ostracized, and it used to bother me, in time, I
learned to deal with and accept it. I suppose supporting evidence could
be found for any belief, but it's my journey, and I get to say what helps

me feel better. I found the perspective of Robert Schwartz quite helpful in living with my decision. He says that,

> *A common plan at this time in history is for souls who want to learn about unity consciousness – the Oneness of all beings – to incarnate into families in which they are very different from all other family members. The interpersonal frictions and even ostracism that result cause them to feel separate. The pain of feeling separation drives them inward, and over time they come into a feeling-knowing of the Divinity that dwells within.*[44]

This viewpoint resonates with me and helps me accept my experiences. I will not say negative experiences because I take them for what they are: just experiences. The only relationships that have had such an impact on me are the ones with my father and brother. The feeling-knowing of the divinity that dwells within not only applies to me but also them. The divinity in me acknowledges the divinity in them, and I thank them for being my most excellent teachers. My experiences with them prompted me to ask the questions and seek the answers to those questions. Was it difficult? Yes! Was it painful? You bet your a$$! However, despite my experiences, or maybe more importantly, because of them, I got to a place of acceptance and love.

It became easy to love them from afar, even though for a long time, I felt negative emotions like hurt, anger, and betrayal. I learned that loving someone, however, does not give them the right to mistreat and disrespect you repeatedly. My journey has taught me about standing up for myself. If it means not having a relationship with them, then so shall it be. I know our physical relationship is through a bloodline, and I believe the more significant, everlasting, and enduring connection we have is a spiritual one.

I will never ask my father, brother, or anyone else to change who they are because I don't like the way they behave. I believe you cannot ask someone to change just to please you. My experiences allow me to live differently than I was before, and for this, I am grateful.

I love and wish for my father all he wants for himself. A few days after Mom's cremation, after all the hullabaloo was over and everybody went back to their corners of the earth, I thought about him and wondered how he handled walking into an empty home at the end of the day. She would put his meal in the microwave when he was on his way home and set the timer. He just had to hit the start button to heat his food when he was ready to eat.

I understood that it doesn't matter how bad things get in a marriage; there is always another being in your presence. To suddenly not have them, it must be difficult. It doesn't matter what you fill your day with or who you see or talk to, when you go home and the person who has been there for more than half your life give or take a few of years, isn't there anymore, it had to be tough.

Even though throughout the years, I believe we had happy times, I viewed our family as dysfunctionally functional. However, the family split down the middle when Mom came to live with William and me, and it got worse as the years went by, even though she returned to her home. As I worked through it, I came to understand that my family dynamics changed when my brother started his deception. My parents were caught in the middle, trying to convince me about his duplicity and not being able to tell him not to do what they suspected he was doing. How could they? Like me, they had no proof. Maybe my father felt he couldn't call my brother out on his behavior; I wondered if he feared he would get the same response Mom did when she tried to talk to her son about his actions.

I presume my father feared he had a lot to lose because he'd experienced being isolated by one of his children and lost the relationship for many years. There were grandchildren now, with the potential of more, and he would have much more to lose this time around. I also contemplated the possibility that my father didn't believe my brother's actions were terrible enough to warrant a conversation and left it at that.

> *There are two ways to be fooled. One is to believe what isn't true;*
> *The other is to refuse to believe what is true.*
> Søren Kierkegaard, Philosopher (1813-1855)

While I was writing and more so, the closer I got to the publishing stage, I became worried about the possibility that my book would cause hurt in my family, or I should say more hurt. I had many moments of doubt about going through with publishing it, one day worried about any negative repercussions and the next remembering the important message I wanted to share.

Then the thought occurred to me; *I was still living in fear*—a fear that manifested when I was a young child. A fear that permeated my adult life and tainted my ability to make healthy choices. I was now fearful of losing what relationships I had left because of what I shared. Part of me was also afraid of bringing shame to my father, thus angering him.

However, I came to terms with it and realized I could no longer allow fear to paralyze me. I've learned that fear keeps you in a kind of bondage that cripples your heart and mind. It poisons every thought, every choice, and every action. It keeps you looking around every corner in your mind for the thing you fear, which creates even more fear, and it makes you constantly hide from your true self. It sometimes feels like being smothered by an invisible force, making it hard to breathe wholly and freely. I had to choose courage and make it bigger than my fear and let the chips fall where they may.

I also thought about how foolish I was for being more concerned about what the truth would do than others who never considered the kind of carnage their lies would possibly cause. It seems everyone in my home myself included, lived in fear of something. I then came across this quote and became more comfortable with sharing my story, without fear or worry that anyone would be hurt because it is not my intention:

> *Better to be hurt by the truth than comforted by a lie.*
> Khaled Hosseini (Best-Selling Author)

I struggled with being so detailed because I told myself that, since I'd dealt with it in therapy with Philip, there was no reason to put it out into the universe. My intuition, however, tells me something different. It tells me that maybe my story could help others to understand their experiences. I kept wondering how any of the pain and hurt will heal if our experiences are consistently covered up and kept as secrets. Others may or may not have the same experiences as I did, but the potential effect is the same; stress, which causes dis-ease in the body that can manifest into diseases.

When I think about it, sometimes it seems as though the pain we cause each other is so ridiculous and undeserved! I try not to necessarily justify every experience I have but rather make sense out of something that seems senseless and hurtful. I believe that every interaction we have with someone, especially when it feels negative, means there is something to learn, and when we learn, we grow. It took a while for me to figure out my potential lesson, and I think learning to stand up for myself was just as crucial as learning forgiveness and compassion. Feeling hurt by the actions of the closest people in my life wounded me to my very core, but it is because of their behavior and my experiences, I am now a stronger person. I am now more mindful of what I will tolerate and accept in relationships and what I will not. It would be so much easier to have a victim mentality, but I think my experiences would have been in vain if I remain blameful and angry, and there would be no growth.

I also consider the possibility that my father and brother each have a spiritual contract with me, for them to learn specific lessons. After all, the fundamental essence of a contract is that both parties gain something from the agreement. I am not the one to know what these may potentially be, because innately, only they would know. I like to believe people see the truth about themselves deep down, even if they have the best façade—one they may genuinely believe at some level. The choice is ultimately theirs to make.

I am even more thankful for my experience with my brother because when I walked away from our business venture, my spiritual journey began as a way to deal with his deception. It was my experience with him that led me to seek and learn the things I've learned; another important outcome is that I wouldn't have met the love of my life, William. Had things worked out differently, I wouldn't even have been in the right country for us to meet the way we did

Regarding Mom's experiences, I wrestled with the idea of sharing them because I knew the humiliation and sadness she felt. Mom's heart was just as broken as her family was, and she felt powerless to put either back together. I can't imagine what it felt like, feeling torn between the lies of one child and the truth of the other! Watching one child hurt the other and powerless to change it must have left her in an emotional minefield, trying to navigate safely between the two. I told her I couldn't have a relationship with someone I didn't trust, and she said she understood, but how devastated she must have felt as a mother?!

To watch your family in broken relationships and to not be able to do what a mother does, nurture it back to health, must have been pure torture. It caused her a kind of pain she didn't know how to deal with, and because she didn't feel she had the support of her husband, it hurt her every day.

In the aptly subtitled section, *The Hurt That Kills*, from his book *The Spontaneous Healing of Belief*, Gregg Braden notes that a growing body of evidence from leading-edge researchers suggests that,

> *'Hurt' can cause the failure of our hearts. Specifically, the **unresolved** negative feelings that underlie chronic hurt. Our beliefs have the power to create the physical conditions that we recognize as cardiovascular disease: tension, inflammation, high blood pressure, and clogged arteries. Modern medicine typically attributes heart conditions to an array of physical and lifestyle factors, ranging from cholesterol and diet to environmental toxins and stress. While these determinants may be accurate on a purely chemical level, they do little to address the actual reason why the conditions exist. What does 'failure of the heart' really mean? Perhaps it's not a coincidence that all the lifestyle factors linked to heart failure are also linked to the force that speaks to the universe itself, human emotion. Is there something that we **feel** over the course of our lives that can lead to the catastrophic failure of the most important organ in the body? The answer is yes.[45]*

After Mom passed, I wanted to know if she'd confided in anyone else about her deepest feelings, and I asked a friend of hers who was more like a sister, as well as a sister, and they didn't know about her deep emotional pain. I was surprised, especially that her friend was unaware of it. Mom didn't have many close friends, and I thought for sure this aunt, who had known Mom since I was a small child, would have known.

That made me a bit sad because everyone should have someone in whom to confide. Later, as I thought about it, I remembered when Mom lived with me, she'd asked me to take her to one of her in-laws for a visit. I got the feeling she needed to talk to someone who was her equal in age, rather than talking to her daughter. I am sure there were things she didn't tell me because, even though I am an adult, I was still her child. I took her but didn't go into the house and told her to call me when she was ready to leave, and I would get her. She made the same request another time, and I took her as she asked, and I did the same thing. I've never asked either aunt what they talked about because I figured it was between Mom and them.

It is important to me then to share what she told me and what I experienced along with her. Maybe by sharing Mom's story, others who are experiencing abuse and, who may feel hopeless, will learn from her experiences; what she did and, more importantly, didn't do, and dare to make a change in their lives. I must say that I don't judge my mother's choices (or my father's or brother's for that matter) as good or bad or that she was right or wrong to feel what she felt. I believe she exercised her divine right to choose; ultimately, it was her right to make the decisions she did.

When I talk about abuse, I talk about not only physical but verbal abuse as well. Schwartz said it succinctly when he wrote that,

> *Statistics about abuse are compiled in a way that creates a false dichotomy. In truth, all verbal abuse is physical abuse. Largely unaware of how energy works, modern society draws an arbitrary and inaccurate distinction between the two. Words are energy, and the energy of abusive words penetrates the chakras of the energy centers, pounding the body as hard as any fist might. There can be no verbal abuse without corresponding physical abuse, even if the effects of the words do not manifest in the body in identifiable ways.*[46]

I thought about Mom's cervical laminectomy, which she needed to take the pressure off of her spinal cord, and remembered Dr. Dean's explanation about the negative impact of stress on the C-spine. I thought about the parallels of both our conditions in this specific area, and I wondered how much of her spinal problem was caused by physical trauma and how much was caused by psychological and emotional trauma. Something caused the issue in her C-spine. Even though we both developed problems in the same areas of our spines, the symptoms we exhibited were unique to our experiences. The one thing that remains constant, however, is the part that stress played as a factor in either case. It is an interesting perspective, one I hadn't thought about until now, three years after I learned about the potential effects of stress on the spine.

I know there is a medical reason for dementia and other diseases, but I also know that our thoughts are catalysts for physiological changes in the body. We are all so unique, with such varying experiences that could result in a myriad of symptoms and dis-ease in the body. Add accidents, environmental factors like pollution, chemicals we knowingly and unknowingly put into our bodies every day, and it's an outright wonder and absolute miracle we are healthy more of the time than we are dis-eased.

One day as I browsed a website catching up on current events, I came across an article about walking depression by Project Helping. I read it because I was feeling so discouraged and wanted to know if I had the condition. As I read the article, it didn't seem to apply to me because the only thing that got me down was the seemingly unending, ever-intensifying pain. If I had even a small bit of relief, I felt my spirit lift, causing a change in my attitude, which made me feel better, and so on. I wondered if Mom could have had this condition, especially in the years leading up to her developing dementia. It always amazed me how she was sad so much of the time, but when she was in others' company, she laughed and had so much fun that no one would ever think she was depressed. I learned that,

> Walking depression is a nickname for the experience of those who are able to go on walking, talking, and even smiling while feeling depressed and profoundly unhappy. The symptoms can

be hard to recognize because they don't fit the more common picture of severe depression, such as someone frequently bursting into tears, gloominess, and lethargy. But it can be just as dangerous to our well-being when left unacknowledged. People who suffer from this type of depression manage to carry out daily tasks and responsibilities, all while suffering from low moods and anxiety. You still get up in the morning, go to work, put on a happy face, and act like everything is okay. And you do so with a general sense of unhappiness.[47]

I really can't say, but I take comfort in the fact that, at least, she was able to laugh and have fun at times. I remembered I did the same when my sisters visited, or when someone called me on the phone, and they were none the wiser to my physical or emotional pain because I didn't let on. I have to believe that Mom had her moments of joy, despite everything. I know it's not my responsibility to make the wish for her, but I do wish she could have experienced more love, compassion, true happiness, and safety within her marriage. I know her experiences are imprinted on her soul, and that her body (and heart), the physical vessel through which she had these experiences, no longer hurts. It is a small comfort.

I also thought about how, from a very young age, I was shushed by Mom whenever I wanted to give my opinion about something. It continued throughout my life, even after I left home when I was eighteen. I knew it was more about keeping peace in the home rather than my opinions not being valid, but it still bothered me. When I read Evette Rose's view on my C1/C2 vertebrae, which is causing the most problems for my nervous system, I can't help but think it's time to speak up and voice my opinions. For most of my life, I did what Mom told me to, which was to keep quiet. As long as her peace and safety were in jeopardy by me speaking my mind, that's what I did. Now that no pain can come to her, I choose to express myself in such a way that others may benefit from my experiences, and Mom's as well.

I feel very strongly that it's not enough just to say I had terrible childhood memories, which impacted my emotional and (most probably) physical well-being. I had to explain what possibly contributed to such dis-ease in my body because it is crucial to understand the effects stress has on the body. Sometimes even with the best of intentions, doing everything we think is right, stress has a sneaky way of affecting our health without us knowing until it is too late. Even worse, sometimes you just don't know what you don't know.

Even though I decided to stop going to the house to visit Mom, I felt so lost because I couldn't see her anymore. One day as I sat to do my meditation, I invited her to join me, spiritually, of course. I imagined her sitting beside me, also meditating, and after doing this consistently for a few days, something began to happen. I started to feel as if she was with me, and I felt such a sense of connection to her that sometimes I found myself smiling. What I felt was so much different from the times we were physically together, and it helped to ease the sense of loss I felt when I made the heart-wrenching decision to give her up.

I started doing the same thing with family members with whom I no longer had contact. I imagined having a group meditation session at my parents' home, and I felt the same sense of connection to them that I felt when I did it with Mom. I couldn't understand the emotion at the time, though, and all I could come up with to explain this feeling was love! I didn't think it was even a tiny bit possible to feel this way again after the experiences I had with my father and brother, but I did.

I understood more the feeling I had when I remembered the inter-connectedness of everything, as Braden explained in the documentary HEAL. He says,

> *We are deeply connected through a phenomenon that is known as entanglement. It's a term in physics that says that once something is unified, once something begins as a whole, even though it is separated physically by many miles or light-years, energetically, everything is still connected. If you go back far enough in time, there was a point where you, me, and the earth were all connected, before what is called the 'Big Bang.' When that happened, physical particles began to separate, but energetically, the particles remained connected. We are part of this earth, and we are part of one another.*[48]

I've read about many experiments that prove this, and I am glad I had the idea as I did my meditation because now I truly feel that all is well. I've heard Dr. Joe Dispenza say memory without the emotional charge is wisdom. I guess I now have wisdom!

I have also changed my perspective about pain, whether physical and most definitely emotional. I believe pain is not an enemy and something to be avoided at all costs, but an indication that something needs healing. The body uses pain to let us know when something is wrong and needs attention. As for emotional pain, it is measurable, and one only has to pay attention to the yucky feeling (emotional charge) in their solar plexus when a thought or memory comes to mind, to know that something is awry. The mere act of suppressing an emotion because it is unpleasant, in itself, speaks volumes.

A word of caution. From my experience, there is no way to get around healing unresolved, long-held emotional pain without more pain. The emotions I felt in my sessions with Philip felt just as traumatic and ago-nizing as when I had initially experienced them. I liken the pain, though, to what it takes to create a beautiful blown-glass sculpture. The glass has to liquefy and endure very high temperatures, and a lot of shaping by the artist. I see pain as the fire, which eventually led to my healing, as unpleas-ant and excruciating as it was.

Mom potentially sought 'forgetfulness' to deal with her emotional pain, but there are a myriad of ways to hide from pain. Drugs, alcohol, work, keeping so busy that you don't have time to think about it, ignoring it, and even religion, sometimes seem like more comfortable ways to deal with unpleasant or painful feelings. We may get relief, but it is only a temporary fix, while the root cause of the pain continues to go unchecked. Using these different means to escape emotional trauma, I feel, is just as ineffective as when the doctors prescribed antidepressants to mask my physical pain.

Emotional pain has many faces: fear, guilt, anger, shame, resentment, regret, hatred, and the list goes on. It is even worse for people like me who think they have dealt with the pain, yet it silently creates mayhem in the body. It doesn't matter which path we take; if we don't deal with emotional pain, the consequence is potentially the same; dis-ease in the body that will eventually result in disease in our bodies.

BELIEVE YOU WILL
FIGURE IT OUT!

For those of you who are going through an experience like I went through, trying to figure out what your body is trying to tell you is wrong and have a diagnosis that does not resonate with you, keep searching! Ask to see the test results. Do the research and **believe** you will find your issue. Don't depend solely on medical doctors because you know your body better than anyone else. We have so much information at our fingertips, and though it may be daunting at times, keep searching. When something makes sense, at least consider the possibilities. Depending on older doctors and believing in their expertise, garnered from years of practice, doesn't necessarily mean they are right, because their many years in the field can potentially result in complacency. Dr. Dean said, "With everything doctors think they know about neurology, they don't know sh!t!" He also included himself in that category.

When you do find the issue, you must keep believing that you will get better, even if it doesn't seem so at the moment. Trust and let your body do what it innately knows how to do, heal itself. Use whatever therapies you believe will assist in your healing, but also be mindful of your thoughts. If you believe even a little that thoughts (conscious or unconscious) can influence dis-ease in the body, then consciously thinking healing thoughts will indeed heal whatever has gone wrong.

If, however, you continue to think the thoughts that potentially resulted in your body becoming dis-eased in the first place, there's a good chance you won't get better. Things can get rather complicated because doctors may discount symptoms as unremarkable, or you may end up in a revolving door of illness and seeking medical attention. We are all unique, and this makes it more challenging. The one thing that became crystal clear because of my experience is how complex, incredibly intelligent, and interconnected the human body is.

For those who are going through emotional pain, which sometimes feels worse than a physical ailment, contemplate the possibility that your emotional pain is part of your (desired) human experience, which may be the driving force in your potential spiritual growth. It is what you do with the emotion that can be life-changing for the better or the opposite. I caution that, if you find that the same emotions keep showing up over and over again, just through different experiences, it may be time to take stock of these and try to understand why.

I am reminded of a 'note from the universe,' that says,

> *Resentment, anger, and impatience all have their place. Actually, they're absolutely priceless, revealing to those who feel them that there are still a few pieces of life's puzzle they've overlooked. They're gifts, like everything else. EVERYTHING else.*[49]

When you do figure out what the physical issue is, I believe it is important also to figure out the potential root cause of the problem instead of only treating the symptom. I don't mean a medical explanation but a metaphysical one. Go beyond the physical symptoms and look at any emotional aspects that may have led to the illness in the first place. Be mindful that you will have to do the work to figure this out because you won't get help from medical doctors. They seem to have drawn an arbitrary line between the emotional, spiritual, and physical body and treat each as a separate entity, one having nothing to do with the other.

As Dr. James said, it is out of their scope because they don't understand it, which isn't to say they can't. There is no excuse not to understand because there is too much information available to continue to live in ignorance. However, their job, if they do it well, is to find what has physically gone wrong and not diagnose patients who trust their expertise with some ambiguous disease while the real issue continues to get worse over time.

My concern is for the young graduates who are interning with doctors like Dr. James. When these kinds of doctors impart their skewed knowledge by training new graduates to misdiagnose patients when they don't understand something, they too will prescribe pharmaceuticals to mask patients' real medical issues. Patients will potentially be caught in a cycle of misdiagnoses while using drugs to deal with pain as one symptom gives way to another, and the original problem remains unresolved.

For doctors who don't understand the mind/body connection, I share Braden's perspective and the science:

The mind/body relationship was documented recently in a landmark study at Duke University, directed by James Blumenthal. He identified "long-term experiences of fear, frustration, anxiety, and disappointment as examples of the kind of heightened negative emotions that are destructive to the heart and put us at risk."[50]

I share one last thought about the power of belief. Through listening to online lectures and speeches by my favorite authors and speakers like Gregg Braden and Bruce Lipton, I learned some remarkable things about the power of belief. For example, there is a story about a medicine-less hospital in China (which is now closed due to political nonsense) where many people were healed without surgery or medicine, from diseases like cancer and heart issues. Their healing probably happened not only because of the assistance of energy healers but more so because they *believed* they would be healed.

I heard Dr. Joe Dispenza talk about the 'spontaneous' healing of participants in group therapy sessions he has all over the world. Sometimes these participants had been plagued with physical or emotional ailments for months and sometimes years. Dr. Joe speaks about the intelligence of the human body to heal itself and how changing one's 'personality' (the way one thinks and feels) creates change in their 'personal reality' (what they live).

There are endless stories about people healing from all sorts of ailments, and they are either considered miracles by some or unexplainable or coincidental by others. However, the scientific community is learning more and more every day by using technology to understand what has been passed down through various religious teachings about belief and healing. The moral of the story, keep believing you will figure it out, and when you do, keep believing you will be healed. And so shall it be done!

EPILOGUE

ubluxation, as defined by chiropractic, is a real thing! If medical doctors continue to dismiss it as hocus pocus or quackery, or whatever they call it, I believe they are doing a great disservice to any of their patients who may have this particular dis-ease in their body. When I first heard the term, I thought it was a mouthful, and it sounded like an easy fix. I learned that was far from the truth for me, and it is taking much longer to get my spine back to its optimal position and performance. When William and I went back to our family doctor after his initial diagnosis, told him what it wasn't (IBS), and used the term upper cervical subluxation, William asked the doctor if he knew what that was. He said no, but he didn't seem interested to find out more. When William explained what my issue was, my doctor's body language didn't convince me that he took it all that seriously.

Our medical system does not work for people like me! If I had cancer, it probably would have been found quickly by the SOC, and the standard treatment protocol would have been applied, depending on my diagnosis. My issues are real, but they were discounted by a plethora of medical doctors and specialists because my symptoms didn't come wrapped in a box tied with a neat little bow. William's faith and perseverance, and his certainty that the doctors were wrong in their diagnoses led us to the answers.

The only way our medical system will change is if more people challenge it, and maybe, just maybe, one day, it will make a difference. Perhaps, one day, doctors will view each patient as a whole entity and stop compartmentalizing medical issues. Their training must have taught them about the interconnectedness of the human body. So they should at least consider the possibility that one strange symptom can relate to another, seemingly stranger one.

I hope I can help others who may be having an experience similar to mine, know that it is possible to get to the answers if you never give up. If this book gives one person the courage and strength to continue on their painful journey, whether it is a physical ailment or emotional turmoil, I count it as a blessing. If one doctor looks at his or her patients as the unique individuals they are, I have accomplished what I set out to do. If one person considers that the experiences in their lives may not be as random as they may seem, and tries to understand the perfection in all of life's experiences; then my journey was worth every second, minute, and hour of pain and frustration. If one person learns that there are many varying perspectives in the world, then I have contributed a bit to humanity, and I offer my humble gratitude for allowing me to share my story.

(At this point, I will ask my readers to forgive me for any boo-boos I may have made in the writing process. There are writing rules, and I tried my best to learn about them, and I hope that the message outshines my errors.) I hope the words written here, with the pure intention of giving hope, find their way to the hearts and souls who need them. I've learned to take it one day at a time, finding comfort and joy in the little things in life, like music, sunshine, flowers, books, or whatever else nourishes my soul. Sometimes when I open my eyes in the morning and feel pain somewhere in my body, reminding me of my human experience, and I feel like giving up, I remember this poster in Dr. Dean's treatment room.

HEALING
TAKES
TIME

You don't get sick overnight
You don't recover overnight
Be patient, you *will* heal

Not the pain, or the relief. Not the answer or the question.
Not the challenge or the victory. The song or the sparrow.
Nothing is random. [51]

ACKNOWLEDGMENTS

My heartfelt gratitude and appreciation for:

Dr. Dean: You have my eternal appreciation for helping me heal my physical body. More than that, you helped me understand what was happening to me when I barely could. I thank you for reminding me that I am more than my physical body and that tending to my emotional health as well as nurturing my soul, were of great importance to my healing. You have my everlasting gratitude for every minute you spent explaining what had physically happened to me, without ever making me feel like I was a bother. My appreciation always!

Tom: Not your ordinary run-of-the-mill physiotherapist! Thank you for putting me on a path to healing I didn't even know I needed. Thank you for finding the anger buried so deep in me; I didn't realize it was there, wreaking its silent destruction. Thank you for introducing me to Philip, and thank you for the first breadcrumb that led to my healing.

Philip: Thank you for your fatherly healing energy! Thank you for helping me heal the little girl who saw things that forever impacted her life! Thank you for teaching me how to go back to her when she needs nurturing and assurance that everything will be alright. Thank you for teaching me that the mind may forget, but the body doesn't. Thank you!

Kathryn: Thank you, my dear sister! Thank you for being there for me! Thank you for always keeping me in the loop about Mom! I have memories of her that were it not for you; I wouldn't have. I appreciate every time you were a pain in my a$$ because I was able to have unforgettable moments with Mom. I appreciate and love you!

Donna: Thank you, my spiritual sister! Thank you for praying with me through the tears in the midst of my giving up. Thank you for reminding me of my true self, the divine consciousness I tried so hard to stifle. Thank you for encouraging me through the process of healing! I appreciate and love you!

Michelle: My Reiki Master Teacher. I was unaware at the time that you did my distant Reiki healing, how much of it was accurate for me. Thank you for teaching me about Reiki, about my true self, about my ability to heal myself, as well as to help others heal, and about living an authentic life free of fear and anger. Reiki blessings to you!

Last but Not Least

I am grateful to all the characters in my story, all the pieces of the puzzle of my life that made the whole beautiful picture I look at today, starting with my father. Thank you for all you did and didn't do for me, and for loving me in your own way. To my brother: I've come into my real power by learning to control my emotional reaction to the things you said, a trait I can now use throughout my life. Thank you for making me strong. Thank you both for helping me on my journey to becoming the person I am today. If we do indeed have spiritual contracts, then you have both done well because I learned things I needed to learn, and *I AM MORE* because of my experiences.

To the doctors who tried their best and did testing to rule out serious medical issues. Thank you! To those doctors who got it wrong. Please! Please! Listen to your patients and don't discount the seemingly 'insignificant' and 'unremarkable.' The diagnosis is in the details, and if you listen with an open mind instead of believing you know everything there is to know about the human body, maybe you will be able to more successfully fulfill the oath you took to help the most vulnerable of people.

My Friesen Press Publishing Team: Thank you for your guidance and for giving me a voice, a voice that has been silent for so long. Special thanks to Alyssa for your insight and vision. The beautiful imagery you created conveys how I felt throughout my journey.

NOTES

1

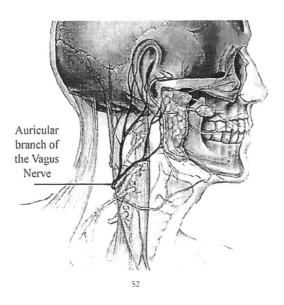

Auricular
branch of
the Vagus
Nerve

52

If there is compression on my vagus nerve and there is a branch that reaches the outer ear, this explains why my outer ear hurt, especially when there was any pressure on it.

2

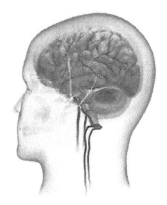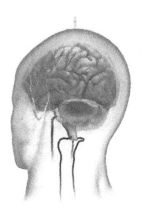

53

These are snapshots of a 3D image showing the reach of the vagus nerve on the surface of the brain. Potentially why I get the sensation as if my brain is vibrating.

[3] The vagus nerve is known as the "wandering nerve" because it has multiple branches that diverge from two thick stems rooted in the cerebellum and brain stem that wander to the lowest viscera of your abdomen touching your heart and most major organs along the way. Vagus means "wandering" in Latin. The words vagabond, vague, and vagrant are all derived from the same Latin root.

In a fascinating new study, researchers at ETH Zurich have identified how "gut instincts" coming up to the brain via the vagus nerve are linked to different responses to fear. The team of scientists was led by Urns Meyer, a researcher and professor (at) Wolfgang Langhans' group at ETH Zurich.

The study is titled "Gut Vagal Afferents Differentially Modulate Innate Anxiety and Learned Fear" and was published on May 21, 2014, in the *Journal of* Neuroscience. The vagus nerve conveys messages between the brain and gut and is constantly sending updated sensory information about the state of the body's organs, "upstream" to your brain via afferent nerves. In fact, 80-90 percent of the nerve fibers in the vagus nerve are dedicated to communicating the state of your viscera up to your brain.

The terms "afferent" and "efferent" typically refer to nerves that lead into or out of the brain. Afferent signals are sent from a nerve receptor into the brain, while efferent signals are sent from the brain to the peripheral body.

Visceral feelings and gut instincts are literally emotional intuitions transferred up to your brain via the vagus nerve. In previous studies, signals from the vagus nerve traveling from the gut to the brain have been linked to modulating mood and distinctive types of fear and anxiety.

As with any mind-body feedback loop, messages also travel "downstream" from your conscious mind through the vagus nerve (via efferent nerves), signaling your organs to create an inner-calm so you can "rest and digest" during times of safety, or to prepare your body for "fight or flight" in dangerous situations.

For this study, the Swiss scientists snipped the afferent nerve fibers of the vagus nerve going from the gut to the brain. Cutting the vagus nerve turned the usual feedback loop between gut instincts and the brain from a two-way communication into a one-way street. This allowed the researchers to hone in on the role that the vagus nerve plays in conveying gut instincts up to the brain.

In particular, the researchers were interested in identifying the link between innate anxiety and conditioned or "learned" fear. In test animals, the brain was still able to send signals down to the stomach, but the brain couldn't receive signals coming up from the stomach.

Healthy vagus nerve communication between your gut and your brain helps to slow you down, like the brakes on your car, by using neurotransmitters such as acetylcholine and GABA. These neurotransmitters literally lower heart rate, blood pressure, and help your heart and organs slow down so that you can "rest and digest."

The Vagus Nerve Is Linked to Fear Conditioning

The new Swiss study explored the consequences of a complete disconnection of signals from the vagus nerve coming up from the gut to the brain, and how this affected innate anxiety, conditioned fear, and subsequent neurochemical changes in the brain.

In a fear-conditioning experiment on rats, the researchers in Zurich linked an unpleasant experience to a specific sound. Interestingly, the gut-instinct signal from the vagus nerve was necessary for unlearning a conditioned response of fear. Through a variety of behavioral studies, the researchers determined that the rats without a fully functioning vagus nerve were less afraid of open spaces and bright lights compared with controlled rats with an intact vagus nerve.

However, without the two-way communication of the vagus nerve between the brain and gut, the rats showed a lower level of innate fear, but a longer retention of learned fear. From this discovery, the researchers concluded that an innate response to fear appears to be influenced significantly by gut-instinct signals sent from the stomach to the brain. This confirms the importance of a healthy vagal tone to maintain grace under pressure and to overcome fear conditioning. The following image demonstrates how extensive and far reaching the vagus nerve is.

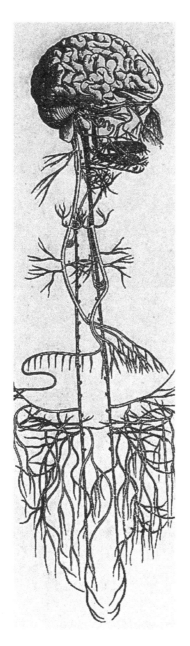

The Vagus Nerve [54]

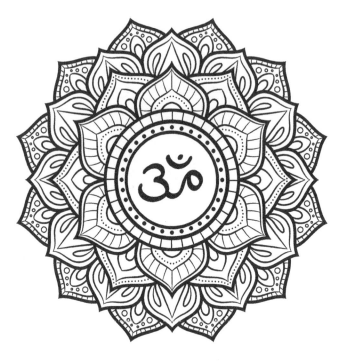

For those who are unfamiliar with chakras: "A chakra is a spinning vortex of biophysical energy or 'Wheel of Light' that absorbs and transmits universal energy in and out of the body. There are seven main chakras, each positioned at specific points along the spine. Each chakra represents a specific gland as well as sub-conscious and conscious states of mind. The chakra system is an integral part in maintaining the overall health and well-being of the mind, body, and spirit, balancing our 'Prana' or Life Force.

The crown chakra (Sanskrit, Sahasrara), is the seventh chakra that sits at the crown of the head. The OM symbol, which sits within a thousand open petals of the lotus flower, depicts the chakra. Its colors are purple or white, and it is symbolic of a higher frequency of energy. The crown chakra is associated with universal energy and spirituality. It is the seat with which one realizes the interconnectedness of all living things. It gives us knowledge and wisdom and enables us to connect with our divinity, becoming one with the whole universe."[55]

1   Wikipedia contributors, "Functional disorder," Wikipedia, The Free Encyclopedia, https://en.wikipedia.org/w/index. php?title=Functional_disorder&oldid=931340158 (accessed July 2, 2019)
2   Dooley, Mike., *A Note from the Universe*, tut.com, December 14, 2015
3   Alzheimer Society, Canada. *Sundowning*. https://alzheimer.ca/en/ Home/Living-with-dementia/Understanding-behaviour/Sundowning (Last Updated:
11/08/2017)
4   Schwartz, Robert, *Your Soul's Gift: The Healing Power of the Life You Planned Before You Were Born*. Whispering Winds Press, 2012. p 33
5   Tolle, Eckhart. *A New Earth, Awakening to Your Life's Purpose*, Penguin Books Ltd., 2005. p139
6   Medscape, *Somatoform Disorder*. https://emedicine.medscape.com/article/
918628-overview, Mar 4, 2014
7   WebMD, *Somatic Symptom and Related Disorders* https://www.webmd.com/mental-health/somatoform-disorders-symptoms-types-treatment#1, 2005-2020
8   Medicine Net, *Medical definition of Subluxation*, Medical Author, William C. Shield Jr., MD, FACP, FACR https://www.medicinenet.com/script/main/art.asp?articlekey=5581, ND
9   Wikipedia contributors, "Subluxation," Wikipedia, The Free Encyclopedia. https://en.wikipedia.org/w/index.php?title=Subluxation&oldid=937269
656 (accessed July 2, 2019).
10   Alternative Care Chiropractic, *What is Thermography*, chiro.org, 1999-2019
11   IAMT (Institute for the Advancement of Medical Thermography). *History of Thermogrpahy*. https://iamtonline.org/history-of-thermography/ #:~:text=The%20roots%20of%20Thermography%2C%20 or%20heat%20differentiation%2C%20are,cold%20temperatures%20on%20the%20surface%20of%20the%20body.
12   NASA. *Thermography*. Judy Corbett. Aug 6, 2017 https://www.nasa.gov/centers/wstf/supporting_capabilities/nondestructive_evaluation/thermography.html

13   MedicalNewsToday, *Everything you need to know about the Vagus Nerve* https://www.medicalnewstoday.com/articles/318128#What-is-the-vagus-nerve (accessed Oct 2018).
14   TermiumPlus, *Osteochondral Bar:* www.btb.termiumplus.gc.ca (accessed Dec 2018).
5   Bing Images, CN X, Vagus Nerve, bing.com/images
16   Spine-health.com, *What is a Physiatrist,* https://www.spine-health.com/treatment/spine-specialists/what-a-physiatrist, September 29, 2011
17   Healthline.com, *Vagus Nerve Anatomy and Function.* https://www.healthline.com/human-body-maps/vagus-nerve, Jill Seladi-Schulman, PhD, August 27, 2018
18   Painter, Frank M., D.C, Wilk v. AMA *25 Years Later: Why It Still Isn't Over,* https://chiro.org/Wilk/
19   AMA Journal of Ethics, *Chiropractic Fight for Survival,* Steve Agocs, DC https://journalofethics.ama-assn.org/article/chiropractics-fight-survival/2011-06#:~:text=The%20AMA%E2%80%99s%20plan%20to%20undermine%20chiropractic%20became%20even,Society%20under%20the%20leadership%20of%20Robert%20B.%20Throckmorton., June 2011
20   Wikipedia contributors, "Parasympathetic nervous system," Wikipedia, The Free Encyclopedia, https://en.wikipedia.org/w/index.php?title=Parasympathetic_nervous_system&oldid=964938471 (accessed July 3, 2020).
21   InnerBody Research, Tim Barkley, PhD., *Nerves of the Leg and Foot* https://www.innerbody.com/anatomy/nervous/leg-foot, July 3, 2018
22   Healthcentral, Beyond Hives: Chronic Neuropathic Itching, Dr. Judi Ebbert https://www.healthcentral.com/article/beyond-hives-chronic-neuropathic-itching, Jan 6, 2017
23   YouTube, *Are Menopausal Symptoms Normal? Think Again! Dr. Eric Berg.* https://www.youtube.com/watch?v=fJ4CX9_soQU&list=PLDdPZKIKxHpM2hYIt5yhwjZojA2T0ZkOR&index=, September 2, 2012
24   Lipton, Bruce., Ph.D., *The Biology of Belief: Unleashing the Power of Consciousness, Matter & Miracles.* Hay House Inc. New York, *2008,* (Location 1186: Kindle)
25   Schwartz, Robert. *Your Soul's Gift: The Healing Power of the Life You Planned Before you were Born* Whispering Winds Press, 2012, p 393
26   International Association of Reiki Profes-

sionals (IARP) January 14, 2020 issue

27   TWE, The Wellness Enterprise, *Dr. Masuro Emoto and Water Consciousness.* https://thewellnessenterprise.com/emoto/

28   Merriam-Webster.com Dictionary, s.v. Metaphysical https://www.merriam-webster.com/dictionary/metaphysical, accessed July 3, 2019

29   Rose, Evette. *Metaphysical Anatomy: Your Body is Talking, Are You Listening?* (Volume One, 2012) 685

30   Rose, 685

31   Rose, 685

32   Rose, 685

33   Rose, 686

34   Rose, 710

35   Rose, 299

36   Schwartz, Robert., *Your Soul's Gift: The Healing Power of the Life You Planned Before You Were Born:* Whispering Winds Press, 2008, p 34

37   Lexico, Powered by Oxford, Meaning of Coincidence, https://www.lexico.com/definition/coincidence

38   Dimension 11:11, *All About Synchronicity,* https://www.dimension1111.com/synchronicity.html

39   YouTube, *Heal Your Body, Mind Whilst You Sleep,* Jason Stephenson https://www.youtube.com/watch?v=4cnU1f1yQR4, April 7, 2018

40   Unite for Her: *Yoga Nidra and the Parasympathetic Nervous System* https://uniteforher.org/2019/12/yoga-nidra-and-the-parasympathetic-nervous-system/, December 2019

41   Wikipedia contributors, "Yoga Nidra," Wikipedia, The Free Encyclopedia, https://en.wikipedia.org/w/index.php?title=Yoga_nidra&oldid=9636813 64 (accessed May 2, 2020).

42   Dooley, Mike., *A Note from the Universe,* tut.com, March 5, 2019

43   Khan, Matt., *Everything is Here to Help You: A Loving Guide to Your Soul's Evolution:* Hay House Inc.2 018, p 19

44   Schwartz, Robert., *Your Soul's Gift: The Healing Power of the Life You Planned Before You Were Born* Whispering Winds Press, 2008, p 48

45   Braden, Gregg., *The Spontaneous Healing of Belief: Shattering the Paradigms of False Limits,* Hay House Inc., New York, 2008, p 110

46   Schwartz, Robert., *Your Soul's Gift: The Healing Power of the Life You Planned Before You Were Born*: Whispering Winds Press, 2008, p 209

47   Project Helping: *Symptoms: Major Depression vs. Walking Depression* https://projecthelping.org/symptoms-major-depression-vs-walking-depression/, July 2016

48   YouTube Movies, (Gregg Braden) *Heal*, Kelly Noonan Gores, The Orchard Entertainment, 2017

49   Dooley, Mike., *A Note from the Universe*, tut.com, April 30, 2019

50   Braden, Gregg., *The Spontaneous Healing of Belief: Shattering the Paradigms of False Limits*, Hay House Inc. New York, 2008, 110-111

51   Dooley, Mike., *A Note from the Universe*, tut.com, December 12, 2019

52   Daith Piercing, *The Vagus Nerve in 3D* (Powered by Biodigital) https://daith.co.uk/pages/what-is-the-vagusnerve, ND

53   Daith Piercing, *The Vagus Nerve in 3D*

54   Phycology Today: *How Does the Vagus Nerve Conduct Gut Instincts to the Brain*: https://www.psychologytoday.com/ca/blog/the-athletes-way/201405/how-does-the-vagus-nerve-convey-gut-instincts-the-brain, May 23, 2014

55   Crystal Earth Spirit, *Crown Chakra*, https://crystalearthspirit.com/pages/what-is-a-chakra, 2020

BIBLIOGRAPHY

Books

Braden, Gregg. *The Spontaneous Healing of Belief: Shattering the Paradigms of False Limits*, Hay House Inc., New York, 2008

Kahn, Matt. *Everything is Here to Help You: A Loving Guide to Your Soul's Evolution.* Hay House Inc. 2018

Lipton, Bruce. H. Ph.D. *The Biology of Belief: Unleashing the Power of Consciousness, Matter & Miracles.* Hay House Inc. New York, 2008

Rose, Evette. *Metaphysical Anatomy: Your Body is Talking, Are You Listening?* Volume One, 2012.

Schwartz, Robert. *Your Soul's Gift: The Healing Power of the Life You Planned Before You Were Born:* Whispering Winds Press, 2012

Schwartz, Robert. *Your Soul's Plan: Discovering the Real Meaning of the Life You Planned Before You Were Born*, Frog Books, 2009

Tolle, Eckhart. *A New Earth: Awakening to Your Life's Purpose.* New York: Penguin, 2008

Van Praagh, James. *Adventures of the Soul: Journeys through the Physical and Spiritual Dimensions:* Hay House Inc., New York, 2014

Songs

Adele, *Don't You Remember,* Album 21, Written by Adele and Dan Wilson. Produced by Rick Rubin, 2011

Dion, Celine. *Because You Loved Me*, Writer, Diane Warren, Producer David Foster, 1996

Urban, Keith. Underwood, Carrie. *The Fighter*, Album: Ripcord, co-writers/co-producers Urban & busbee, 2017

Websites

Alternative Care Chiropractic, *What is Thermography*, https://chiro.org/acc/

Alzheimer Society Canada: *Sundowning* https://alzheimer.ca

AMA Journal of Ethics, *Chiropractic Fight for Survival*, Steve Agocs, DC, https://journalofethics.ama-assn.org

Bing.com: *Vagus Cranial Nerve Branches*: https://www.bing.com/

Dimension11:11. *All About Synchronicity*. https://www.dimension1111.com

Dooley, Mike. *A Note from the Universe*. tut.com

Health Central: *Beyond Hives: Chronic Neuropathic Itching*, https://www.healthcentral.com

Healthline: *Vagus Nerve Anatomy and Function* https://www.healthline.com

Innerbody: *Nerves of the Leg and Foot* https://www.innerbody.com

International Association of Reiki Professionals: IARP.ORG

Lexico. Powered by Oxford: *Meaning of Coincidence* https://www.lexico.com

Medical News Today: *Everything you need to know about the Vagus Nerve* https://www.medicalnewstoday.com

Medscape: *Somatoform Disorder* https://emedicine.medscape.com

Merriam-Webster Dictionary, *Meaning of Metaphysical* https://www.merriam-webster.com

NASA, *Thermography*. https://www.nasa.gov/centers/wstf/supporting_capabilities/nondestructive_evaluation/thermography.html

Phycology Today: *How Does the Vagus Nerve Conduct Gut Instincts to the Brain*, https://www.psychologytoday.com

Project Helping: Symptoms: *Major Depression vs. Walking Depression* https://projecthelping.org

Termium Plus: *Osteochondral Bar.* www.btb.termiumplus.gc.ca

WebMD: *Somatic Symptom and Related Disorders*: https://www.webmd.com

Wikipedia: Functional Disorder

Pelvic Splanchnic Nerves

Parasympathetic nervous system

https://en.wikipedia.org

Videos

Noonan Gores, Kelly. Documentary: *HEAL*, 2017

Stephenson, Jason. *HEAL Your Body Mind, Whilst You Sleep - POWER of Focused Desire (Guided Meditation)* April 2018

YouTube, Dr. Eric Berg. *Are Menopausal Symptoms Normal? Think Again!* https://www.youtube.com/

YouTube, *The Power Of Thoughts, Words, & Intention- Masaru Emoto's Experiments With Water*, https://www.youtube.com/

YouTube: Dr. Masaru Emoto's Water Experiment - *Words are Alive!* YouTube.com